Still of Darkness

Still of Darkness

By Bill Coakley

ISBN-10: 1941142060

ISBN-13: 978-1-941142-06-6

Published with the help of JETLAUNCH www.jetlaunch.net

Contents

Dedications:

Anne Marie Fontana. You are my love, and my life. We were on top of the world when you passed away at the age of 26. We will be together again in the blink of an eye.

Also for my Mother and Father, who have passed and waiting on the other side.

Last but not least, all the wonderful partners and co-workers I have had the privilege to work with over the years— keep the faith. I sleep soundly at night knowing Police, Fire, and ambulance are a phone call away.

For information on publicity contact:

Brian Sawyer Vice President @ billcoakley.com

Buzz Sawyer Marketing/Sales @ billcoakley.com

Acknowledgements

Chris and Debbie at JETLAUNCH, who made this book possible.

Best-selling author Echo Heron for her wonderful insight and help.

Best- selling Amazon author Ruth McLeod for her wisdom and help— I'm looking forward to the next book!

Still of Darkness

CHAPTER ONE

3:00 am Jan 21, 1986

As the loud and high-pitched tones sounded through the cold darkness of early morning, I awoke startled and disoriented. Where was I? The thumping in my chest gave way to clearer thinking as the loud and high-pitched tones sounded a second time. With my eyes suddenly open, I was surrounded by the complete and still of darkness. I quickly realized I was in Arnold, on my last 24-hour shift as my pager crackled out, "Medic 64– Code 3 traffic."

At this particular time, working on the ambulance meant 24-hour shifts and a 72-hour work week. That was considered the normal for EMS (emergency medical services). I liked to stack my shifts together, so I always ran 72 hours straight at my full-time job for Riggs Ambulance in Merced. It made you numb to the calls, and everything would simply turn into a blur. And trust me, working for Riggs in the 80's meant ambulance duties as well as coroner service, so numbness, along with a foggy blur of sleeplessness, was a very welcome feeling. While I've been told that laws exist to discourage the transportation of the dead to the morgue in an ambulance, Riggs Ambulance Service had a sacred contract with the county to provide coroner services, and as such, we on the front lines were often dispatched to deliver the dead. So, off we went about the business of transporting the deceased, toe tags were used for identification after rolling into the county's always-arms open and awaiting morgue. An extra-large, walk-in refrigerated locker was used to stack corpses, young and old, onto the cold, stainless steel cots. Of course when you are new, you think it's all really fun and interesting.

However, that wears off quickly. Especially after working your ass off trying to save a cardiac arrest patient, who doesn't survive. You write your report, clean and restock your ambulance, so that you can finally head back to quarters, only to hear the pager blasting those thoughts into oblivion as you are now being ordered to return to the hospital and transport your last patient to the morgue. We saw every death that came in, from infants to the elderly, from the sick to trauma-related, high-speed roll-overs, stabbings, and shootings. Three of the hundreds of dead still come very vividly to my mind.

A middle-aged male whom had last been seen alive a week earlier, was found in his second-story apartment bedroom. When we walked into his residence, and before being greeted by the bloated and incontinent body, we could smell death mixed with heat and humidity. The lack of ventilation made it hard to describe with mere words. The patient looked to weigh in at a blubbery 350 pounds or more, which would be a good catch for a yellow fin tuna, but not so good for us. We wrapped the corpse in multiple sheets and blankets to help with the stench and oozing body fluids, and then strapped him onto a backboard. With both of us pulling, we inched our corpse to the top of the outside stairs, and then kind of rode him toboggan-style to the bottom of the stairway. Hey, send the paramedics to do a four man coroner's job and that is how it gets done.

Another case that is forever scorched into my subconscious, only to come out during restless sleep, is a call involving a self-inflicted gunshot wound. When we arrived to the rural area with a circular dirt turnout, a single vehicle sat under a very large and old oak tree. We heard the song "Stairway to Heaven" blasting from the car, which we later found out to be set up on a portable dual cassette player that played the song over and over. When we stepped out of the ambulance, it was a warm summer morning and the two sheriff deputies that were on-scene, hastily retreated from the vehicle where the victim had managed to scatter his brains. The gunshot wound took off the top of his cranium, but left skin tissue draping over the bottom portion of the skull, an eerie sight I must admit. This particular year Riggs had allowed us to wear blue cargo shorts and Hi Tech Mountain boots with our Riggs Ambulance white polo shirts, which was awesome in the sweltering heat of the central valley. We were also the envy of all the other ambulance personal from other companies who were sweating their asses off. We were freshly showered and ready to start the day in our new summer uniforms. We had just started heading for breakfast when we caught this call, which certainly was not going to be a great way to start the day. The victim had somehow managed to get the barrel of his shotgun into his mouth and successfully pull the trigger, not an easy feat. We grabbed two body bags: one for the victim, and one for the scattered skull and brains. Steve Buckingham, better known as Buck or Bucky, was my partner that day. Bucky was as twisted, or even more so than I, as he shouted with glee when he found and pulled a piece of perfectly clean skull out of the car's interior ceiling. Later, after delivery to the county facility, we headed out for breakfast which would be for one of our favorites, machaca and eggs found at one of our many frequented Mexican restaurants. Often we would go an entire 72-hour shift eating only Mexican food, which was far from friendly when in close quarters. We were digging into the chips and salsa and awaiting our machaca (which is scrambled eggs mixed with beef, bell peppers, and onion, served with rice and beans, and of course corn tortillas) of which we made ourselves several breakfast burritos. Bucky suddenly had a sly grin on his face, reached into his pocket, and slid the piece of skull he dug out of the cars ceiling across the table to me. Bucky was always trying to up the ante on gross and unthinkable actions to help lighten an otherwise sick and twisted world. It was always crazy working with Steve, as you learned to become hardened to all the exposure of death and dying, you took on a laugh-at-it-all attitude to keep it all from spilling out.

The third dead patient I can never seem to erase from memory, was when were responded for a human briquette. Shovels in hand, we went into to the freshly burned mobile home. The fire department had gone home after the blaze was put out, which left just us to search. Water was dripping from the charcoaled ceiling above, spattering on our backs and necks and onto our once-clean jump suits. The patient was a thirteen year-old male, or so we were told. He looked more like a piece of burnt furniture than anything else. One body, one bag, thank you and goodnight. In the morning, I would wake up confused as to where I was, and then realize I had four days off in a row. This was indeed very wonderful, just like a mini vacation every week.

Not today, however, as the pager repeated: "Medic- 64 Code 3 traffic" for the second time. Every other week I pulled a 48 on Medic 64 for the Pucch in Arnold. Why I picked up this part-time gig with Joe Puccio at Calaveras Ambulance was not reasoning well with me at the moment, especially as the blond beside me rolled over and sleepily tried to pull me back into bed. I slid out of the warmth of the bed, grabbed my jumpsuit from a peg on the wall, and zipped myself in. I then stepped into my black leather zip-up Red Wing boots when my worst fear was confirmed. The Pucch's eight year old son announced over the radio, "Medic 64, respond to Bear Valley for a medical aid."

Oh well, I've had better days. And as far as paramedic jobs went, there was the free skiing at Bear Valley, the free membership at Kline's gym, and of course the mountain cabin where we were stationed. Also, nobody treated a paramedic with more respect or bragged more about his employees than The Pucch. Hell, he would promise to pay you next week, and then buy you breakfast instead. Money was tight, but Joe was the best boss ever. Anyway, if I wasn't here, there wouldn't be a paramedic to work this side of the county for the next two days. This was 1986 and Calaveras County had just increased their level of pre-hospital transport services to paramedic in 1984, which also happened to be my first year as a new paramedic.

It would be a solid 3 ½ to 4-hour round trip call if all went well, as I wondered what the weather forecast might be. Starting down the stairs from the loft and glancing at the sleeping blonde one last time, I found Brian just stepping out of his room, yawning and lighting a Marlboro at the same time. Brian looked at me and said, "I've been up here for six days and need to get home. I told Joe I had to be off today." "Yea, buddy, not a problem. Drive like hell and when we get on scene we will limit our time with the patient to ten minutes or less and haul ass out of there." Then another thought occurs to me. Let's hope the

Pucch's card works for fuel this time. I think my partner paid for it the last time, as the card was refused.

Chapter 2

2:45 am Jan. 21, 1986

Dr. Zawacki was also asleep when his pager went off and awoke him in the early hours of the morning. He had a good day of skiing while on one of his regular, but far and few between, vacations to his cabin in Bear. As always, upon his arrival he had checked in at the first aid station at the bottom of Bear Valley's ski runs, and been given a radio and pager as an available emergency physician during his stay. This was not a paid position it was a service from the heart. Dr. Ken Zawacki became a permanent fixture at the first aid station, often never even getting a chance to throw on his skis and make a run.

Back at the station, Brian stubbed out his cigarette and we both started grabbing gear to tote down to the unit. In the winter, we brought the medications and a complement of IV solutions inside, because the drugs and IV solutions would otherwise freeze at this temperature and altitude. The engine block was plugged in to keep it warm. Joe had tried many times to install small portable heaters for the back of the unit to heat the gear, but they kept blowing fuses. So down the side of the cabin and to the unit we went carrying bags of gear and a 747 Plaino box, which is a large fishing tackle box that found its way into early ambulance use, and, in my opinion, was the best and easiest to use.

The Pucch came over the radio, broadcasting that we were responding to a seven year old boy who was unresponsive and that the patient and family will be at the first aid station. "10-4 copy," replied Brian, who then looked at me and said we were going to be rolling into some big overtime. I laughed back as we both knew we were probably going to catch a free breakfast, along with a promise to be paid in a few weeks. We finally arrived, turned the unit around in the snow-covered parking lot, and drove backward, toward the first aid station's ambulance parking /loading dock. We got out of the ambulance, slipping and sliding to the back doors, throwing all the equipment we might need on the gurney, and pulled it out. Wheeling a gurney through slush and ice is not nearly as scary as the possibility of stepping into potholes that are filled with frigged slush and water, since that would make us miserable for the next several hours. As we rolled into the first aid station, which would normally be closed at this hour, we get our first glimpse at the seven year-old boy on a hospital bed with his parents standing over him.

He was on oxygen via a nasal cannula, and he had been hooked up to an ancient EKG machine (probably donated thirty years earlier). We also noticed an IV of D-5 and half NS had already been started (sweet, less work for us). Now, we just needed to move quickly in here and get back on the road. As we rolled our gurney alongside the hospital bed and nod at the parents, Dr. Z comes over with a warm smile and says, "Hey it's good to see you two up here." I gave the Z a quick handshake as he took me aside to fill me in on the patient's condition and medical history. It's always nice to see a familiar face and, in Zawacki's case, we had worked together for several years off-and-on. While pouring a cup of coffee, Dr. Zawacki told me that the family noticed their son acting a little strangely the last few days, while on their skiing vacation. Early this morning, they saw him tumble down the last to steps of inside stairway, and now he was not conversing. The family stated that there was no PMH (past medical history) or medications, which of course should rule out diabetes, seizures, etc. There was no evidence of alcohol and the patient's parents were also prescription medication-free. Doctor Z, while limited to x-ray equipment and simple cardiac arrest drugs, had already performed an x-ray and ruled out any spinal fractures. I replied, "Interesting case; what do you think? Head trauma, tumor, or maybe meningitis?" The Doc took a sip of his own coffee and stated that the patient's pupils were equal and reactive, his reflexes were intact, and that the child had no fever. The patient, while currently nonverbal, moved both sides equally, which ruled out pretty much any type of cerebral vascular event, but then again, not necessarily. Of course, there was always the chance that he got into somebody else's medication. Dr. Zawacki told me that this was pretty serious. The patient needed a full workup as soon as possible, and I needed to keep a close eye on his airway while transporting him. As we transferred the patient, James, over to our gurney, I glanced at his last set of vital signs: blood pressure was 102/62, heart rate was 110 (a little fast, but not serious), and respirations of 24 per minute. Because the patient was a minor, the mother was going to ride with us (up front of course). I usually do not take family members along because if things go south they have a way of adding to the difficulties. In this case, however, I did not have much of a choice since James was only 13. Brian would keep her occupied up front. Out into the cold, early morning we went with light snow flakes beginning to fall. After loading the patient into the ambulance, I leaned forward to Brian and asked him to start Medi-Flight. "Tell them we are westbound on Hwy 4 from Bear Valley and we will meet them." Brian complied, and after radioing in he stated that they were attempting to lift off from Modesto, but the weather was touch and go. I acknowledged, "That's why I want them. In case this storm gets worse, and we get forced to chain up." The patient's mother was belted in the front passenger seat and keeps looking into the back where her son is next to me, on the gurney. The mother asked Brian over and over why she cannot be in the back. Brian, one of the best partners and friends a guy could ever have, was skilled at explaining that everything was fine and continually changed the subject from "What exactly happened" and "Had this happened before?, to "How many children do you have?" I reassessed James' vitals and, most importantly, his level of consciousness.

Normally if you speak to a patient and they answer coherently, you can assume they are alert and oriented. If they do not speak, then applying a reasonable degree of pain through various methods is the next step to generate and assess a response. I generally start with a soft sternal rub that increases to the point that a patient attempting to fake unconsciousness will scream, spit, and fight. If painful stimuli is not successful, then a gag reflex is next on the list. Without a gag reflex, the patient is at risk of airway compromise, and the airway can become blocked by the patients tongue, as well as the patient may vomit and aspirate (which would be like drowning). After a very strong sternal rub with no response, I will check a patient's airway with an OPA (oropharyngeal airway), which is a curved piece of plastic that comes in different sizes to accommodate patients of all ages and sizes. It will keep the tongue from sliding back and obstructing the airway, but it is not a help if the patient vomits or needs to have his respirations assisted. Intubation (placing an endotracheal tube into the trachea) is the king of all airway protection.

I spoke to James, asking him to open his eyes with no response. I started off with an increasing sternal rub without reaction. I rechecked his pupils, which were equal and reactive. As I watched him breathe, I noticed that his respirations were becoming more rapid and deep. Something clicked in my brain, so I leaned forward and smelled the patient's exhaled breath and realized it was fruity and acidotic, just like the textbook description for diabetic ketoacidosis (which is called hyperglycemia or more simply put high sugar).

In ninety-nine out of one hundred medical aids for diabetics, the patient is hypoglycemic (low sugar) from having taken their insulin, but also being extra active or not eating, causing a generally rapid decrease in level of consciousness. The simple fix would be a glucose paste from a tube if the patient is still conscious enough to maintain their own airway or 25 grams of D-50 IV Push for an adult if the patient has no gag reflex. If you cannot get an IV, you can inject Glucagon IM (Glucagon is a hormone that stimulates the liver to release glycogen). James, if my diagnosis was correct, might be a first-time onset of diabetes, where the pancreas is not able to release the insulin needed to transport the glucose molecules to the cells, which leaves the body unable to metabolize the sugars and it turns to metabolizing fats. The brain, however, needs glucose to function, the initial onset of diabetes is generally slow, over days to weeks of increasing thirst and frequency of urination and mild to moderate dehydration.

Ordinarily, patients that we pick up who are unconscious and unresponsive and who have no known medical history would receive Narcan and D-50. Narcan is an anti-opiate and the D-50 is glucose or simpler, sugar and water. In the 1980's, we did not have glucometers. So if the patient was a known diabetic, we would use a wonderful litmus paper strip that tested if their sugar was either high or low.

So instead of blindly administering D-50 and Narcan to every patient who did not respond, we would take into account their medical history and the medications they were taking. For example, an elderly patient of 75 years-old, found to not be responding by family members, would first be ascertained if they were diabetic or not. Without a diabetic history, along with no noted hypoglycemic medications, checking their pupils for the pinpoint tell-tale of a narcotic overdose, and further coupled without decreasing respirations, we could rule out diabetes and narcotic overdose and move on.

Being a good paramedic means being a good investigator, so when the 75 year old does not speak and only moves one arm towards pain full stimuli, it begins to look like a possible CVA or hopefully a TIA for the patient. A CVA or cerebral vascular accident is considered a dry stroke caused by micro emboli breaking free (usually from the carotid arteries) and becoming lodged in smaller arteries of the brain. A TIA or transient ischemic attack is similar, but only temporary as the micro emboli manage to dissolve by themselves.

With all this in mind, it did not make sense to consider James' condition to be a diabetic emergency, especially with no history from the parents. I knew that the helicopter would appreciate two IV lines, so I set up a bag of normal saline, tore some plastic tape, and grabbed an 18-gauge catheter, followed by laying out a litmus paper. I missed the first IV—which is never good because you are now stuck with damage control before trying again. I did, however, get a drop of blood on the litmus paper and low, or not-so-low and behold, James' blood sugar was off the chart, high. After controlling the bleeding I had started, I managed to get the next 18-gauge in proper placement. I replaced the original D-5 and half N.S. with a second bag of

Normal Saline and noted the total fluids infused so far. Brian was doing his best to get us down the hill before the storm hit and we lost our window of opportunity to utilize the bird and got further regressed to putting on chains. Brian leaned over and told me that the first landing zone at Big Trees State Park has been cancelled due to the current weather forecast, and the next landing zone would be Arnold. The patient's EKG was beginning to get more rapid with lots of ectopic beats, so I opted for a 20cc per kg. fluid bolus, which calculated to about 100cc's. No help. I began to think about metabolic acidosis and realize that, while not in our paramedic protocols for this type of case, maybe Sodium Bicarbonate could be of use. I fully realized that the patient, James, was in need of insulin, which we did not carry. Sodium Bicarbonate, at the time, was still primarily for use in cardiac arrests and also for tricyclic overdoses, as well as anti-cholinergic exposure. I am not one to ever ring the base and ask for orders, but in this case, I was not one hundred percent sure. I attempted base contact, hoping to confer with a physician, but the med-net radio was not getting out. Unable to reach the hospital, I decided to see if James had a gag reflex. He accepted the OPA without objection, so I decided it would be safest to protect his airway and hyperventilate him in order to help with the acidosis. I did the math for pediatric endotracheal tube sizes and came out with 6.0, which is the first un-cuffed size. I managed to slide the patients tongue to the left with the laryngoscope blade. I waited and watched while his vocal cords opened and closed and timed it just right as I placed the tube a few centimeters past the vocal cords.

There were no end tidal CO2 detectors, or esophageal bulbs, and certainly no capanograpy on the ambulance to verify proper intubation placement at this time. So, after visualizing the placement, you looked for fogging in the tube and listened to abdominal and lung sounds, followed, next, by assisting ventilations and watching for even chest rise and fall. With the endotracheal tube in the correct position, I used a syringe to inflate the pilot balloon with 10ccs of air and secure the tube in place. I was then assisting respirations at 26-30/minute, nice and deep, and more regular than the patient's own breathing. There was no notable change in blood pressure, just a concerning irregularity and increasing of the boy's heart rate. I was not certain what possible rhythm to expect, as this was never taught during my paramedic education. Brian called me up front and gave me the news that the landing zone in Arnold has been pulled as well, and the helicopter would now attempt to land in Murphy's, which was right off Hwy 4 at Sierra Construction's football field-sized parking lot.

Brian whispered that we just passed a "chains required" sign for uphill traffic, and that The Pucch had been updating him on the company radio that the snow level was supposed to drop in the next hour and hit Angles Camp at the 1,400-foot elevation (which was rare) and Murphy's, our new destination, was at about 2,400 feet in elevation. So, tell me the good news, Little Brother. That was Brian's nickname that went back to a call when we picked up one of our many patients, who were under the influence of alcohol. When we had arrived on scene for the intoxicated patient, for whom I have zero tolerance, Brian stopped me before I could jump out and start in with a verbal assault on the patient, who was of course, lying next to a dumpster across from a liquor store. Brian put his hand on my chest and told me to stay put—he's got it. By the time we got to the hospital, the patient and Brian are chatting it up like old pals. We put him in the back room as a low-priority and far enough away from the nurse's station to not attack their olfactory senses. As we were leaving the room, Brian handed him a twenty dollar bill and the guy saluted Brian and yelled, "Little Brother, I love you man!" Brian made sure to tell the nurse to treat him extra well, while I was doing my best to not shake my head "no" and choke Brian out. Before I could do this, he added in that if there were any problems to call him personally and gave the nurse his phone number. Outside, Brian told me the story of how the drunk was one of six survivors from a mission in Vietnam of the 101st Air Borne. Brian continues, "Every year since returning home, they have met together. Today was that anniversary, and he was all that is left." Personally, I have picked the guy up more times than I can recall for being drunk, but Brian, being Ex-Navy, has a weakness for military patients, so be it.

The good news, Little Brother told me while driving through the falling snow down the highway, is that the flight crew was allowed to, and did, lift off and are now landed in Murphy's, awaiting our arrival. He further stated that they can only hold for five minutes, as foul weather is approaching. "OK, Little Brother, give it all you go". It looked like we were still a good ten minutes out, so I told Brian: "In five minutes, confirm we have a visual on them, and ask them to hold for another five minutes more, as we are rolling in." As the storm chased us down the winding pine tree-lined highway, the Medi-Flight helicopter came into our foggy and drizzling view. When we pulled into the parking lot, the normal procedure of the crew coming on board the ambulance to get a patient history and reassess vitals and procedures, is cut short to a quick wave towards the hot landed bird. A hot landing is when the helicopters blades are rotating and the engine is ready for flight. We handed off James with a quick explanation and promised to radio a med-net report to Memorial North Hospital as soon as we got

back in our rig. Brian is explaining to the mother that her son is going to Memorial Medical Center, and the helicopter of course does not have room for her. About that time the husband in his Ford Ranger slid into the parking lot as the helicopter was lifting away, the husband and wife hurriedly drove off with the directions we had given them. A week later, we received a thank-you letter from the family, stating that James, while now a diabetic, is fine.

CHAPTER THREE

I was currently living in Angles Camp and, when not working my regular shifts in Merced, I would do standby for The Pucch, who lived about three blocks away. The Pucch, who currently could not afford to pay me, would put my time on the books if he did not have any other paramedic coverage; of course knowing that if I did not step up, there would be no paramedic service for the city. Calaveras County, at that time, had increased their level to paramedic, but did not require the ambulance providers to have a paramedic onboard. Many of the ambulance services were still basic EMT-level or paramedic when they could find one. When The Pucch could not staff a paramedic in Arnold, we would roll up Highway 4 to meet with the BLS unit (basic life support). Joe would usually pick me up if the call was North of town or up Highway 4. If the call was South of town, we would meet at the bank on Main Street.

The Pucch's wife was also an EMT and, on this particular day Joe was out of town, I was covering with his wife, Charlene. Charlene was extremely friendly, but had no desire, in fact absolutely hated, anything to do with the ambulance. How she ever obtained her EMT is beyond me. The phone rang, and when I answered, Charlene told me that we had a call at New Malone's Lake in the Glory Hole boat-launching area.

I knew the area well, as I had worked six years for Tuolumne County Boat Patrol as an officer. I attended Modesto Junior College, taking the PC 832 class (which equates to a level 3 officer trained in laws of arrest and gun handling) which is the minimum requirement to operate alone and with a weapon. We patrolled Don Pedro Reservoir, Tulloch Lake, Pinecrest Lake, and New Melone's Lake. There were three full-time employees and three part-time deputies, of which I was the newest. My first encounter with a dead body came one night when fellow officer, Jay Coates, called me at home at approximately 9 p.m., stating that a jumper went off the Archi Stevonot Bridge (about a 130-foot drop) into New Melone's. He was excited and asked if I would come with him to search the area by boat. It sounded like an adventure to me, so off I went to meet him at the office and hook up a patrol boat. Jay was nervous that Calaveras County Boat Patrol would get there first, as half the lake was in each county. By the time we reached the boat launch on the Tuolumne County-side of the lake, it was quiet and dark. There was deepness and stillness to the dark black water, and the sky above us sparkled with stars. When we launched our patrol boat, Jay drove as I worked the spotlight out and over the lake as we approached the bridge. No sign of any other boats on the lake, and no traffic on the bridge above. Jay had told me, as we drove to the lake, that a driver saw a woman jump from the bridge and called it in. CHP had found an abandoned vehicle on the side of the road next to the bridge, and a women's hand-written suicide note inside. I figured the chances of finding anything were next to none. As I played the high-intensity spotlight back and forth seeing nothing, Jay started screaming "Over there, over there!" Floating in the dark waters ahead of us I could just make out a small object floating. As we slowly motored forward, the small shape became that of a woman's back, in dark clothing, bobbing in the gentle and still water. We tried three times to bring her aboard, almost to the point of tipping and/or falling out of the boat to no avail. We secured her lifeless body to a rope and tied it off to the boats starboard side cleats, and slowly boated towards the shore with our catch. When we released our prize from our jerry rigged roping, she reminded me of a big rat with her arms half-bent and stiff and her jaw clenched solid with teeth snarling. I was feeling some kind of adrenaline pumping and an acute sensitivity of hearing and sight, like being out on the edge of a cliff, pumping through my veins.

When we had enough man-power to double up on patrol, my regular partner was Rick Rutherford. He was an ex-Seal Beach Policeman and the surfer type, who taught me a lot about the job and then some. When Rick was driving the patrol boat, which he always did, it was hang on or fall out. I told him one day, "If we crash this thing and I die, you will lose your job." Rick said, "Nope, I will stick your dead ass behind the wheel and go home early." One holiday weekend as the crowds swelled out of the city towards the mountains and lakes, we decided to put two boats on Lake Tulloch. It had three bars and since lots of alcohol and fast boats don't mix, we thought it best to play it safe on our end. As the afternoon sun was beginning to set, we were called out for a medical aid; a water skier had dislocated his knee. There were four of us in two patrol boats. One officer had taken the Advanced First Aid course, another officer was an EMT, and the third officer outranked me, so my job was to stay offshore and slow incoming boaters down so their wakes would not cause turbulence. The others were helping the patient and preparing him for transport into our patrol boat. We would then meet with the ambulance that was en-route to the South Shore boat-launching facility. It was this particular event that sent me down the path to becoming a paramedic. I considered the shifts I had patrolled on several of the large lakes alone, and decided I needed some medical training. Emergency Medical Technician training is a one-semester college course, and at the time it was being offered at Columbia Junior College. I signed up for the class after being told by others that it would be wiser to take the Advanced First Aid class first, as preparation. I figured it couldn't be that tough and I could handle it. I had no idea that there were 206 six bones in a human body and that they all had names. Learning about a pneumothorax and a life-threatening tension pneumothorax, where a paramedic can do a needle decompression is what led me to learn more. Back to college for some anatomy and physiology and EKG interpretation, and then to paramedic school, I went.

In 1973, Stanislaus County, where I attended school, became the second county in California to have a paramedic program. Going through the program ten years later, I had the opportunity to meet, and work with, many paramedics from the original classes. We were also one of the few areas allowed to intubate pediatrics and perform nasal intubation. I had done my paramedic training in Modesto and Turlock, and started off as a new medic in Calaveras County in 1984. I later worked three years in Merced and Mariposa counties for Riggs Ambulance, followed by a full-time position in 1989 at Turlock Ambulance. The Stanislaus Paramedic Class of 1983/84 was still free of charge when I went through it, except for the books. Since there weren't any paramedic text books written yet for the earlier programs, we had six telephone book-size medical books to lug around. There were also no pre-paramedic classes, unlike today where a student will take a general combined class on anatomy and physiology, as well as EKG interpretation. We were stuck with college-level anatomy and physiology, which included cadaver's centrifuges and trays of separated bones, in which we had to identify each and every tubercle and fossa. The college EKG class was even more fun, since they had not learned to start students with a simple, straight forward interpretation of rhythms. That is where Dubbin's EKG book came in. It was basically the *EKGs for Dummies* of its time. The only other big difference in old-school paramedics was that when we did our field time, we had one year to get signed off by three field training officers, and while there was a minimum amount of hours spent per person, anything after midnight did not count. For the most part, it took about of a year of interning in the field before being set free.

Two summers earlier, in June of 1984, just prior to formal graduation from paramedic school, I was working the lake with my friend and co-mentor, Officer Rick Rutherford. It was the weekend of Mountain Aire at the Angles Camp fairgrounds. Music worshipers were invading the area as Rick and I refueled the patrol boat at the dock and chatted with Pappy, who was about 85 years old, well-weathered, and a salt-of-the-Earth from Arkansas. Pappy owned a very small and simple houseboat; he also ran the fueling station for a minimal, under-the-counter fee agreement and free docking. About the time Rick and I were done conversing with Pappy about how well his crawdad traps were working with canned cat food as bait, up the dock walked Ben Orr, the lead singer/guitarist of the Cars. He was strolling down the boat launch as simple and average as the rest of us, absolutely not identified by any guests at the resort. He introduced himself and told us he was here for the Mountain Aire Concert. He later said a helicopter would be picking them up in the morning to fly the band members into the Angels Camp Fairgrounds. Pappy, with a twisted and unbelieving grin on face, disappeared into his houseboat and came out smiling and holding a small Casio Keyboard. About the same time, another average-looking guy, by the name of Greg

Hawkes (the keyboardist for the band), was looking for his pal Ben. Greg was enjoying a beer as he stepped onto Pappy's porch. Pappy disappeared, again, into his old houseboat to retrieve an old, beat to hell and back, loose-stringed guitar. Ben took the guitar from Pappy, Greg picked up the keyboard, and the fun began. Rick promised to show up in the morning and handle any crowd control for the band, when the helicopter came in to transport them to the concert. Rick had showed up as promised and ended up getting a helicopter ride with the band to the Angels Camp fairgrounds, where he hung out backstage and met most of the other musicians. He called me in the early afternoon to pick him up at the fairgrounds and bring him to Lake Tulloch for our late afternoon shift. Lake Tulloch, with its three bars and dozens of pumped up jet boats and v-drives, was always crazy on the weekends. Rick always carried a Walther PPK as his service weapon, and I carried a Smith and Wesson model 19 357 with two sets of speed loaders on my belt.

The sun was starting to set, and we were in the patrol boat at the Poker Flat area, when we heard the sound of loud, uncorked headers, on a jet boat barreling past us. Hmmm, this could be good. The driver of the boat is traveling too fast to be safe, so we slowly start after him to see what he will do next. The driver of boat, who is clearly attempting to set a new Tulloch Lake speed record or is just plain crazy, drives the boat, full-speed, into the base of the mountain. This was beginning to look interesting. When we pulled up, the boat was sinking and he was in the water hanging onto the boat. We pulled alongside of him carefully, to help him aboard the patrol boat, but he shouted at us to get the hell away. We told him the obvious, "Your boat Is sinking, get on board." He yelled, "No, I am staying with my boat." Two of his friends in another boat pulled up and threw him a rope, and at this point it looked like the boat was going down like the Titanic with only about one foot of the nose sticking up horizontally. His friends were towing him with a rope as he hanged onto the tip of the bow. The Poker Flat Marina was about one hundred yards away, so we figured they would attempt to pull in there. No, he refused our orders to pull into the Poker Flat Marina, as well as the order to put on a life jacket. Instead, he insisted on going approximately two miles further to the launch at South Shore. I looked at Rick. He shook his head and stated we would follow and save his ass if it looked like he may drown. Somehow, they managed to get him, and the 99% of the sunken boat, to the other launch. He held the rope, while somehow managing to tow the sunken boat, for almost an hour, still refusing to wear a life vest. After arriving at the South Shore ramp and walking out of the water, we promptly arrested him for reckless and dangerous operation of his boat, along with being under the influence. We were not out on the lake to ruin anybody's day, and would have gladly helped him into our boat and towed his boat to the closest marina, while letting him off with a stiff warning, except he failed the attitude test, and brought the arrest on himself. It was just another day of the usually calm shifts on the lakes with the occasional drunks, and even more occasional drowning. One of the funny things about boating laws is that while water skiing, the flagger has to be a minimum of twelve years of age. How to ascertain this is tough, however, since twelve year-olds do not have driver's licenses. The interesting thing is that there is no age limit on the *driver* of the boat, which means an eight year-old could drive the boat, but is unable to be a flagger. We kept this to ourselves, along with the fact that you can operate a boat while drinking, but you cannot be under the influence of alcohol.

Charlene called me back after I noticed she had not arrived at my house, and it had been five minutes since she first called. "Where are you?" she asked. I told her "Joe always picks me up if the call is North of town." She replied "sorry, can you meet me here?" "No problem, I am on my way," when I arrived, she was in front of the ambulance waiting for me, stating that the unit would not start.

I tried all of the several accessory switches and low and behold if the ambulance was not dead. I pulled my truck up and popped both hoods in an attempt to resuscitate the ambulance. I placed jumper cables on both batteries. It would be fruitless to try and call for another ambulance from a different provider to take the call as the next closest unit is twenty minutes away. The ambulance roared to life, and I dropped both hoods and pulled my truck out of the way. Into the now rumbling Medic 62 unit we went. Of course, it is about a thirty minute drive to the Glory Hole access boat launch and while Charlene is driving code 3 in the left lane, cars were passing us in the right lane. The only thing that is worse than driving to a call too fast is driving too slowly. When the call came in, it was for a 75 year-old male complaining of chest pain while out fishing on a boat. When we arrived on scene at the boat launch area, the volunteer fire department was doing CPR. As I grabbed for the Life Pack 5 (cardiac monitor and defibrillator) and the Plaino tackle box that has all of the airway tools and medications, Charlene decided to head over and relieve the fire department of compressions. Holy mother of shit, I should have never answered the phone. Having to drive up to The Pucch's house, jump start the ambulance five minutes after receiving the call, and then driving in slow motion to the scene, now I didn't have a partner to direct, because somehow she decided to think on her own. "Charlene!" I shouted as I was walking towards the would-be angler, "Let the fire department continue CPR. I need you to place the patient on the monitor and then set me up a line of Normal Saline solution." This should keep her busy until my next orders. I obtained the medical history from the patient's fishing partner, and I'm told that the patient, John, had been having indigestion before breakfast and it continued after arriving at the lake. They had been fishing for several hours when John turned pale and grabbed his chest. By the time they got to the ramp, he was not breathing. His friend also told me, that as far as he knew the patient had no medical problems and took no medication. I wondered to myself if I should ask if they had any luck out fishing. However, I realized my sense of humor might not be appreciated. With the EKG connected, I asked the fire guys to hold compressions while I checked for a rhythm. "Asytole, flat line, no good, continue compressions, you are all doing a great job."

Sliding the patients tongue back with a Miller number 4 attached to the laryngoscope, I managed the 8.0 endotracheal tube two to three centimeters past the vocal cords. I watched for equal rise and fall of the chest during ventilation and auscultations over the abdomen first, then both sides of the chest to confirm proper tube placement. I now aggressively secured the ET (endotracheal tube) tube in place with cloth tape. I knew that the prognosis was grave (and that the patient probably had "the big one"), but I continued on, administering 1mg of Epinephrine followed by 1mg of atropine down the tube. John's rhythm was still flat, despite doing a routine check of the different leads on the monitor and double-checking that everything was correctly placed. The next step was starting the IV for which my partner had set up, "Thanks Charlene. Tear me some plastic tape for the IV then pull the gurney out of the unit and bring a backboard over here." I grabbed a 14ga angio catheter and turned the patients head to the right and slid the large catheter into his left external jugular vein with a red flash into the catheter's chamber, identifying that my placement was good. I put another round of Epi and Atropine through the IV line that was wide open and I hoped for a miracle that was not going to happen. Once in the ambulance, it was a tragically slow ride to Mark Twain Hospital, Firemen were doing compressions and ventilating, while I fruitlessly pushed Epinephrine every three to five minutes and topped out on my max dose of Atropine at three milligrams. I tried Sodium Bicarbonate and Calcium Chloride, and even threw in some Dextrose 50 percent and Narcan. The once full ambulance cabinets were being depleted of medications and the empty medication boxes were strewn everywhere. When we arrived at the hospital and entered the emergency room, it took less than one minute for the ER physician to call the code and mark the time of death.

CHAPTER FOUR

Two days after the fishing expedition at New Melone's Lake and I was back at home, asleep, when the phone rang. I opened my eyes and cleared my head. It was 1:00 am in Angels Camp when I picked up the phone. I heard Joe saying, "Motor vehicle accident. Hwy 4, west of town, toward Copperopolis." "Ok, I will meet you at the bank. You buying breakfast?" "Of course, anything you want. Let's do this." It sounds like a good one; East of Copper, in the Dead Man Curves. The Dead Man Curves have long since been straightened out, but not before they provided Calaveras Ambulance with much-needed working capital and payroll in the 1980's. Pucch was pulling into the abandoned bank parking lot as I jumped out of my truck. I stepped into Medic-62 who, with her pale blue body and dark blue stripes, was the mirror image of her sister, Medic-64 in Arnold. The difference is that 62 was Joe's baby, and she had a mildly aggressive cam and headers, a 750 Holly double pumper carburetor, and, of course, it was the only ambulance I knew of with two separate sirens. What beautiful music you could sustain, running code 3 down Main Street on a warm summer's day. The Pucch, with his two lazy eyes, Grecian Formula hair, and pants falling down his backside whenever he bent over, was an absolute magician with the radios. It was a wonder how he could manage to haul-ass code 3 with two radio mikes on his lap, changing from one to the other with two conversations at once. He would have the Calaveras Sheriff on one and the hospital or CDF on the other, speaking fluently back and forth, while adjusting the wail and yelp of the two sirens and sliding around the highway curves. Joe told me the call is for a car that ran, head–on, into a tree. It happened on the infamous curvy section of West Highway 4, and fire and highway patrol have been dispatched. The Pucch came alive on code 3 runs, and I caught a little adrenaline rush, myself. It's almost like a rollercoaster just reaching its peak and getting ready to fall. The Pucch asked if I wanted Medi-Flight, and I said, "Sure why not? Maybe we will catch a hot Flight Medic or Flight Nurse. Bring them on." While simultaneously talking on both radios, Joe explains to me that the two-fold beauty of the helicopter is this: Number one, He got reimbursed 80% of his ambulance fees from Medi-Flight and that was great, because he got paid whether the patient was insured or not. And number two, we could be back and available to run calls, make money, and maybe even save a life. Medic-62 was the only ambulance I knew of that actually had a "We accept Visa" sticker on the back window. The Pucch has the carbon paper triplicate charge sheets and the impress slider in the unit. If you could get a patient or family member to pay with their credit card, they would get a 10% discount on the day of the transport and you would get a free dinner at Perko's Café, compliments of Joe. It may sound unprofessional, but Calaveras Ambulance (Joe) was struggling to make ends meet, and Joe did treat his employees well.

With lights flashing in the darkness, we continued our code 3 travel down the highway towards Copperopolis, which was, among other things, home to the Poker Flat Resort. It had boat launching facilities, a large hotel with a restaurant, and a bar all on the lake. Shaking my head and rubbing my eyes, I focused back on the deadly curves of the highway coming up fast. We were first to arrive on scene with Copper Volunteer Fire rolling in next, followed somewhat later by CHP. There were two patients: a driver and a passenger in a midsized car. It was located just off the road and pushed halfway into an oak tree with the hood crumpled forward and the windshield starred on the driver's side. There was no significant interior vehicle damage, even though the exterior's impact is major. The driver was male, approximately thirty years of age, and the passenger a female, whom appeared about the same age. I approached the driver and started my assessment by asking him what happened. "I don't know. Where am I?" he replied. "Do you hurt anywhere? What is your name? What was the last thing you remember?" I asked. "I don't hurt at all, my name is Jack, and the last thing I remember is leaving Copperopolis and heading for home in Angels. What happened?" While talking to him, I instructed him to not move his neck. A firefighter got into the back seat to maintain the patient's C-Spine and placed a cervical collar on the patient. I had introduced myself as a paramedic and told him that my name was Bill. While taking a nice strong and regular radial pulse and noticing a hematoma on his forehead, I asked the fire department to extricate the patient on to a backboard to get some vital signs and told them I would be right back. I spoke with Joe, who has assessed the second patient and told me she probably had a fractured femur. I grabbed the Hare Traction Splint just in case she did, and then headed in her direction. The fire department reported that their second unit was setting up a landing zone about a mile away, in a church parking lot. As I worked my way over to the second patient, I told Joe that the driver would be patient number 1 and would be first to go. Joe jumped into the driver seat of his baby Medic-64, and started wielding both radios at once, reporting to the sheriff's department on one frequency and updating Medi-Flight on the other. He also updated the local hospital, Mark Twain, for good measure. I was in a quandary while I examined the freshly-extricated Janet from the wreckage, thinking to myself that I cannot leave with the first patient to fly him out and leave the second patient unattended. I am the only paramedic on scene, and we are not allowed to release our patients to a lower or less trained level of care. Joe stepped beside me and answered that question for me by telling me that he had arranged for both birds, Medi-fight out of Modesto and Cal-Star from Sacramento, to land at the L.Z. at the same time.

The second patient, Janet, was in a lot of pain and trying to hold back her tears. Since it appeared to be an isolated injury, I had Joe set me up a line of Normal Saline and retrieve a 1cc syringe and 10mg morphine for the patient. Doing a secondary exam and cutting clothing away to evaluate possible wounds, I found that she did have an obvious left femur fracture, and there was also considerable swelling in the left thigh. Checking pedal pulses on both feet to make sure there is no circulatory compromise, I found good, equal pulses and slowly begin pulling traction on the left leg. I pulled the leg with manual traction and the patient was moaning, but said it felt better. I had a firefighter take over the manual traction as I prepared and fit the Hare Traction splint that would maintain traction at whatever level was most comfortable. With the splint strapped on and cranked into the appropriate position, I rechecked her distal pedal pulse at the left foot and I was greeted with a strong and steady pulse. While The Pucch set up the first IV, I initiated a 16ga angio catheter in the patient's right antecubital and taped it in place. The vitals given to me to by the volunteer firemen were good with a blood pressure of 128/70, a pulse of 80 per minute, and respirations of 18 per minute. After confirming that our patient had no allergies, I explained to her that I was going to administer 5mg of morphine. I told her that she may feel a little woozy or nauseated and to let me know if she thought she may get sick. The Pucch and the firemen had

Jack out and on the gurney at the back of the unit. As the volunteers and I carried Janet over, we placed her onto the back bench in the unit. When we loaded Jack in, I began working my way between them. Both patients had been placed on oxygen, and Joe had a second IV line set up for me to start on James. We left to meet the helicopters and I was told it should be about a five minute drive. I did a third hands-on assessment on both patients and another set of vital signs for each; nothing had changed. I placed three electrodes on each patient and hooked up the leads to Jack first, and then Janet. I was not expecting anything abnormal on the patients EKGs, but it was another precaution to rule out any irregular rhythms. Irregular rhythms can sometimes be caused by blunt trauma to the chest, causing a cardiac contusion. Both patients were in normal sinus rhythms, so I prepared to get an IV going in James. In trauma, bigger is better. So a 14ga easily goes into Jacks large rope-like vein in his left upper arm. We were almost done when Janet started moaning in pain again, so I delivered the rest of the pre-drawn Morphine as we pulled into the church parking lot. As I looked up to the vast darkness of the early morning sky, I saw the beautiful sight of two medical helicopters that were surrounded by the flashing lights of fire trucks, CHP, and firemen pointing their flashlights and directing orders back and forth like a symphony being led by a conductor. We gave report on the two patients to the Flight Medics and headed back up highway 4 toward Angels. Joe was excited and happy about us using the helicopters. That was also my first time using two birds simultaneously. It went extremely smoothly, and I appreciated the ease with which our patients were transferred.

On a different motor vehicle accident two weeks later up Hwy 4 out of Angels on the Utica grade. Two vehicles had struck head-on before sliding down an embankment and coming to rest two hundred yards from each other. I was working Angles Camp with another paramedic and when we went en-route, we called the Arnold BLS unit to come in for extra help. The Arnold unit got there just after we did and we radioed for them to take the first vehicle. We ended up extricating all the patients and I got switched to handle the other vehicle, whose patients were already loaded in the BLS ambulance. Charlene was driving and I jumped into the back. An off-duty female paramedic named Robin had stopped to help and was in the back of the unit when I climbed in. I asked her, "What do we have?" She said Joe had told her that these were her patients and that I should set her up an IV of Lactated Ringers, she was going to start an IV on a four year-old male that was complaining of abdominal pain. I asked what his vital signs were, and she responded that she did not have any yet, and then reminded me again that Joe told her these were her patients. I realized there were a lot of patient assessments and vitals to be taken and I had no time to deal with who was in charge. I simply stuck my head up front and told Charlene, "The next wide spot you see in the road, go ahead and pull over." Charlene pulled over and I told Robin, "Out. Now." She got out and I left her on Hwy 4 between Murphy's and Angles Camp. She was yelling that I would not get away with this. I did.

It was not fun making that decision, but there was no time for discussing who was in control, and you certainly don't start IVs before you have fully assessed your patients. There were four patients, two of whom were set up on hanging cots, one above the gurney and the other above the bench seat. There was just too much to be done. She also had the four year-old in position number 3, on a hanging cot, above patient number 1, who was on the gurney. This was not the proper placement for a child, especially when he/she was potentially more injured than the other patients.

As two years roll by with the numerous medical aids and even more numerous drunks and system abusers, I found myself working in Los Banos, a city in the western part of Merced County. Los Banos is a windy city just off Hwy 5 with lots of agriculture farming and a population of about 33,000 that particular year. Getting the Los Banos shift is done by seniority, since medics tend to want the smaller cities with less call volume. The rural area also generates more potential for serious medical aids and fatal motor vehicle accidents. A winning combination as it is not the quantity, but the quality that makes running ambulance exciting. Ron Duran was the resident EMT and my partner for the 72-hour stints in Banos. The crew's quarters are a hospital room at Los Banos Community Hospital, but if their patient status rose and they needed the room we are in, we would make accommodations at the Bonanza Motel in the center of town. In over a year of working with Ron we never stayed at the hospital. We always stayed at the motel with continental breakfast and a swimming pool. Of course, being resident EMT and the one who daily called in the hospital's patient status to dispatch, Ron had control over where we quartered up for the shift. For a paramedic, working out of a motel was definitely a perk, along with better high-end calls and less call volume. Ron and I had worked together in the windy city all summer, slowly gaining trust and respect among the police department, fire department, and hospital staff. I remembered my first day working with Ron, whose nickname among close friends was "Little Duck" from his surfing days in South Mission Beach. That first day, Ron told me, before introducing me to the hospital staff, that the charge nurse was a royal bitch to ambulance personnel and to stay clear of her. As we made our rounds through the Emergency Room and started towards the floor, we ran into the charge nurse who immediately wanted to know what we were doing on that floor: who authorized it and why. I looked at her, then at Ron. Before he could reply, I asked if they had any coffee. With a confused look, she pointed and said it is in the break room. I replied, "I like mine with one cream and one sugar, how about you, Ron?" The nurse shook her head and walked away. Ron, a little bit concerned about pissing her off, learned lesson number one in patient and co-agency verbal interactions: if you are nice to me, I am nice to you, and if you are rude to me, I will up the stakes. I had to explain to him that we don't work for the hospital and we never give quarters in a verbal assault. I knew that for her to complain about me asking for a cup of coffee would make her look inadequate in the face of her peers. We never had another problem with her after that, and Ron soon realized that when working with me on Medic 91, we took no prisoners. The summer rolled on with the usual chest pains, diabetics, seizures, and CVAs, along with an occasional high-speed roll over and ejection or pin-in.

On October 12th, we were fast asleep in the Bonanza Motel when the high-pitched sound of our pagers went off, beckoning us to duty. A vehicle in the Delta-Mendota Aqueduct, twenty miles out, toward Hwy 5. "Copy. Medic 91 en-route." It sounded as if it might be a decent call. We listened to our scanner, picking up CHP and fire department traffic, stating that a vehicle had gone off the road, into the canal, and sank. Unknown injuries. Driving Code 3 and talking with dispatch at the same time, Little Duck hammered down on the throttle as the information update told us there was a possible of five victims, three of whom are children. Arriving on scene, we saw two adults, who appeared to be a husband and wife, standing next to a CHP cruiser. A fireman with a high-intensity light searched the large aqueduct. After ascertaining that the couple is ok and requesting another ambulance for them, the couple told us that the car lost control and went off the bridge. They had three children unaccounted for, ages 1, 4, and 7.

Ron and I, along with two firemen, scaled a locked gate onto a dirt access road that ran along the aqueduct. Three hundred feet from the gate, we saw the headlights of the submerged car eerily glowing through the deep water. We were unable to see the car, because of the poor visibility offered by both the darkness and cold, moving canal water. The firemen were searching the water with two high-intensity lights that both stopped on an object in the area of the headlights that was indiscernible. The Little Duck and I looked at each other and the only question was: you or me? Ron had a minor cold with cough the last week, so the decision was that I would go and he will come back with the ambulance and more help to get me out after searching the area. I took off my radio and pager, followed by belt, shirt, and lastly my Red Wings, and I slid down the embankment and into the water. The two firemen were keeping the area lit for me as I began swimming in the cold water. I would never recommend this type of rescue to anyone, since if you, yourself, get in trouble, it can make everything else worse. However, if there was going to be any chance of recovering a life, this was it. It was now or not at all. As I swam toward the area where the firemen were shining their lights, I felt a strong surge of current, which certainly gained my respect. The water was cold and dark, and I noticed that the undercurrent was stronger than I expected as I reached the area of dimmed car lights. I found myself in the middle of the aqueduct, and looking ahead, I saw the shape of something floating just in front of me. I reached for what later turned out to be the seven year-old girl floating, face down. I grabbed her and could not feel any breathing or pulse, so I gave a few quick rescue breaths. I swam as strongly as I could on my left side with her head up, under my right arm. As I reached the steep side of the aqueduct, there were at least six firemen and my partner who were tied off on a rope that Ron had hastily wrapped around the axle of the ambulance. I realized that without them, there was no way I could physically get the girl out of the water, let alone myself. Later, Ron told me that when he reached the ambulance to get more help, he asked if the CHP Officer could open the gate. The officer told him that he was not about to open the gate, so Ron said to the officer, "My partner is in the aqueduct trying to save a patient, and if you do not open the gate, then I will simply run it down with the ambulance." The officer immediately unlocked the gate. Arms grabbed me as I passed the girl up the human chain of firemen, belayed to the rope. When the patient was passed to Ron, he placed her on a backboard and started CPR. A cervical collar was placed and the young girl was strapped to the board. I felt that while the odds were small, we would run this like a trauma code and drowning combined. The monitor was attached and showed a PEA (pulseless electrical activity) 86 bpm (beats per minute) which simply means there was a rhythm without a pulse. This is normally not associated with a good outcome, however there are times with a PEA that the heart is functioning and we just cannot detect it. We will hope that is the case.

Other causes of PEA, which are taught in ACLS (advanced cardiac life support) (high-end CPR for doctors, nurses, and paramedics), include shocking, medications, intubation, and circular reasoning. These are all reasons as to why the patient may be in any given rhythm at any certain time. In the case of PEA, you would consider the mnemonic of the H's and T's (H's are hyper or hypokalemia, hydrogen based acid, heroin overdose, hypovolemia, and hypothermia, and the T's are tamponade cardiac, tension pneumothorax, toxins, and thrombosis).

At this point, I was considering the obvious, which is trauma, drowning, and hypothermia. I managed with some degree of difficulty to intubate the patient with a 6.0 endotracheal tube. I watched the chest rise and fall, while auscultating over the abdominal area and then both lungs. The tube was good and it was now secured with cloth tape, .8mg of Epinephrine 1:10,000 down the tube, and I started looking for an IV site. The Duck had already prepared the IV line and torn me some plastic tape to secure it in place, before jumping up front and heading to the hospital code 3, I had one fireman doing compressions and another ventilating the patient. The first attempt for an IV was a miss, with little collateral damage as far as bleeding was concerned. The second attempt was good, however it is only a 20ga catheter and while I opened it wide, it is slow. Attaching a blood pressure cuff around the IV bag and pumping it up helped the flow considerably. More Epinephrine was administered through the IV line, and that would be repeated every three to five minutes. We had the heater on in the back of the ambulance and several warm blankets on the patient where we could. I was dripping wet from head to toe with no shirt on as we arrived at Los Banos Community Hospital. I stomped my wet, bare feet into my leather boots, and out of the ambulance and into the ER we went. The whole staff was awaiting us, and I could see that we all really wanted to save this young child. I was shivering as I gave the report to the emergency room physician; Ron had called in the basics over ten minutes ago. Little Duck handed me a towel and placed a warm hospital blanket around my shoulders as I continued my report. The hospital staff was going all out when they got a pulse and faint blood pressure. The x-ray staff was coming in with their portable machine, while the doctor was making arrangements to fly the patient out. When the x-rays came back about ten minutes later, the patient had lost pulses and CPR was started again with more epinephrine. The doctor looked at the x-ray images and pointed out several cervical spine fractures, one being at the C-1 level and is not connected to the brain stem. All efforts were stopped and our hopes would be for another day. The Little Duck and I have gained some more respect and trust from the hospital staff and fire department, however to save the little girl is all that we wanted.

As we put the unit put back together, we were asked to respond back the accident scene, pick up the other two deceased children, and transport them to the Los Banos Mortuary. The Los Banos Search and Rescue Team had utilized scuba divers and a tow truck to pull up the sunken vehicle, in which the four year-old boy had been trapped. The other child, a one year old infant girl had been recovered floating down past the bridge. We loaded the deceased children into the back of the ambulance and we were up on the aqueducts single-lane dirt embankment. We could not turn around and had to drive miles to find a spot where we could get off the Delta-Mendota dirt road. Why I was driving was beyond me, as everyone knows I get lost. And I did. After driving thirty minutes in the middle of nowhere, I pulled up to the first intersection, read the names of the two streets, and got out the map. Meanwhile, Riggs dispatch is calling us to find out where we were and what is taking so long. The two street names were not on our map book. We were heading towards a small, unincorporated town named Firebaugh that was not on our map. Finally figuring out the correct direction, I decided it was best to have Ron drive us. We continued to ignore the dispatchers on the radio and turned off our headlights as we passed another ambulance that was posting for us between Los Banos and Dos Palos. When we arrived at the mortuary, we were greeted by two females, about our age, who ran the place. They had a coffin for a coffee table, and wanted to know if we had ever had sex in a coffin. They told us they had prepared a twenty-four year-old girl for her funeral earlier that day, and asked if we wanted to see her. I looked at Ron, and we got the hell out of there.

Chapter 5

Riggs Ambulance Service, while in Merced County, also covered Mariposa County, which consists of Coulterville and Mariposa. One ambulance in each town, Coulterville was the least-populated of the two, and another good place to get some rest and run fewer calls. We were currently stationed out of the CDF fire station where we had our own room with bunks and a restroom. The unit sat in front of the third fire department bay, which was empty inside. We took our meals with the CDF crews, who numbered about ten to twelve firefighters at any given time, and we cleaned up the kitchen with them after meals. At about 5 p.m. in the summer, we would play some serious volleyball into dinner time and often continue after dinner for another hour or so.

On duty and asleep, at the CDF station we awoke to the loud beep, beep, beep of our pagers and radios coming alive. Sitting up in bed and putting it all together (like where I was), I reached for my jumpsuit and stepped into it. I saw Brian doing the same, only faster, and I knew he would be out to the ambulance first to light up a cigarette. As we jumped into the rig and started it up, the dispatch center notified us that we were responding to a male with a rattlesnake bite. Brian seemed a little nervous, so while driving to the call code 3, I asked him how to handle a rattle snake bite. He started off on a disarray of snakes, poisonous venoms, and treatments. It was unexpected and showed that he was very knowledgeable on the topic. When we arrived on scene, we found a thirty-five year old male who had been drinking heavily. While trying to catch the snake, he was bitten in the left forearm. The patient was acting tough in front of his friends by telling us that he did not need an ambulance and to go away. I simply deferred to the sheriff officer present, who told him, "Ambulance, or jail for intoxication?" It was the ambulance for the soon-to-be not so tough guy. Once in the ambulance, he asked me if this was bad and I simply told him, that he might not make to the hospital in time. "What, are you kidding me?" "No. You might die from this—sit still and do not move your arm." I placed a tourniquet above and below the bite just loose enough to place a finger under, I then circled the bite with a felt pen and noted the time. Little Brother has set me one IV bag of Lactated Ringers Solution and wrote the patients vitals and the time on the pillow slip for me. I asked Brian for an easy code 3 to Sonora Community Hospital, and I would do the rest en-route as we had a 45 minute drive ahead of us.

Placing the patient on oxygen at 4 liters via nasal cannula and hooking up the three lead monitor, I prepared for an IV. I don't want the IV on the affected arm, so I dropped a 16ga into his right AC, connected the IV tubing, and secured it with tape. "What are you doing that for, are you serious?" the patient blurted out, "yes I am serious; let me know if you get a metallic taste in your mouth." "What do you mean? Why?" "Let's just say it gives me an idea of how much time we still have." Which it did not, but the guy was still acting like an idiot, so that was how I would treat him. Of course, there are many factors involved with a pit viper bite, such as how much if any venom was released and where the bite is (the extremities being of a better outcome than a more central bite). The venom can cause hemodialysis with acute renal failure, and the patient could further go into shock. I decided to start a second IV in the right hand to be safe. The swelling in the patients left arm was increasing, and as he sobered up, he was starting to get rightfully scared. After spiking the second IV line with Lactated Ringers Solution and placing a 16ga angio catheter in the patient's right arm, a car nearly clipped us as it passed, going the same direction on the highway 49 curves to Sonora. Brian quickly got on the radio to dispatch to advise CHP. He picked up speed to get the plate number and better description of the make and model. Snake bite guy was hanging on to the gurney tightly as Little Brother slid around the twisty two-lane highway. After catching up and writing down the plate number and a brief description of the vehicle, Brian took a deep breath and called it in to dispatch. The dispatchers stated that CHP was up ahead and waiting for the vehicle, and we should hit the siren as we passed if that was the car in question. Up ahead, at the bottom of Old Priests Grade, CHP had the racer pulled over, and Brian hit the siren twice to confirm the identity. Our patient is now extremely concerned as his right lower arm is now twice its normal size. It was time to radio the hospital and give a med-net that would apprise them of our ETA, and current patient condition. We were still about ten minutes out as Little Brother continued our code 3 quest for the Sonora hospital. The patient's vital signs had remained stable during transport, and his earlier laughter had turned into occasional tears. When we arrived at Sonora Community Hospital, we were greeted by Doctor Bill Stiers and emergency room physician Rob Lyons, who appeared to be enchanted by the somewhat occasional rattlesnake bite. The nurses prepared the anti-venom while I filled the two physicians in on the call, the approximate time the bite occurred, and no, I did not bring the snake in, and yes, it was a diamondback rattler. The anti-venom is ready, and it was piggy-backed through one of the IVs on the patient's right arm. The doctor called for an in-house surgeon since the left arm was now almost three times its normal size and it caused what is known as compartment syndrome. The arm must be basically filleted open to keep all the swelling from cutting off circulation and causing the patient to lose his arm. It was no laughing matter. The patient was looking at a minimum of a three-day stay in the hospital to let the hospital monitor his condition. It was time to head back to the CDF station in Coulterville with another story under our belts.

The first call I ever ran with Brian was out of "Hooterville", as most of us indigenous to Coulterville called it. The 911 call was for a twenty year-old female having seizures. Brian was pretty new and, in fact, he only had an ambulance driver's license (which was the law's minimum requirement, and it gave you one year to complete EMT training). At this point I was a 5-year medic, just starting to become seasoned, with a lot to still learn on the streets. As we responded up Greely Hill at about 3 am, Brian had the lights going and told me he was going to use the siren as we slid into and out of the dangerous corners. I did not want to say anything since we are new partners, so I just clamped my jaw shut and held on tight. Code 3 with lights and sirens up Greely Hill at 3 am was definitely over doing it. You can only go so fast, and there was no traffic. When we got on-scene at the two story cabin, I jumped out without saying a word to the Brian. I entered the house to find an alert and oriented twenty year-old female who had a history of seizures. She had run out of her medication and was refusing our services. Sounded good to me, "make sure you tell your doctor what happened. Fill your medication and call back

if you need us." Brian finally made it in the door with some kind of medical backpack with an oxygen cylinder inside, strapped on his back. He had the medication bag in his right hand and an airway bag in the left. I looked over at my robo-partner and asked if he brought the clip book because I needed a patient refusal form.

Brian, being the compassionate, unknowing ambulance driver that he is, walked over to the patient, got down on a knee next to her, and proceeded to tell her that this was an emergency and she really needed to go in. I was thinking that I was going to kill my partner. We had a 3-4 hour round trip ahead of us and a patient that would be discharged before we left the hospital. Of course she heeded the medical expertise that my partner had given to her, so I slowly choked my temper in check. When we walked her to the ambulance, which was a good clue that nothing was wrong, I told my new partner to put the patient on a nasal cannula at 4 liters and attach her to the EKG monitor. I figured if I have to transport this patient, there's no better time to assess my new partner's skills. When he was done setting up an IV bag of Normal Saline and tearing tape for me, I told him "Thanks, let's go. We arrived at the emergency room in Sonora, and I was all too familiar with the drill. History of seizures, not taking medication, Okay see your physician, fill your script, and take your medication as stated." The twenty year-old patient was out of the ER before we could restock and clear back to quarters. The thing about seizures is that eventually they all stop. There are many different types, all of which are caused by various disorders, but the majority of seizures are idiopathic, meaning they happen for an unknown reason. Status Epileptics is one actual emergency, since the seizures have not stopped for over ten minutes, or the patient has not regained consciousness before the next seizure begins. The main problem is not so much the seizure, but the muscle of the diaphragm not working; it can cause asphyxia from not being able to breathe. At that point, we simply administer valium to control the seizure and assist respirations as needed.

Chapter 6

I was offered a managerial position from Riggs Ambulance, which meant that I would handle the two Mariposa units if and when the new five-year contract was signed. However, I was later approached by the Mariposa County Medical Director, Dr. Mosher, who wanted me to put in a competitive ambulance service bid for the county. This was no problem because if Riggs got the contract, I was manager for the Mariposa Operations and if not, I got the bid and I am in the ambulance business. Mariposa County provided Riggs with the ambulances and a subsidy to run the service, which was one ambulance in Mariposa and a second one in Coulterville. It did not work out as planned. Riggs won the bid, then fired me for creating competition against my employer. I did not see that one coming. Many co-workers thought I was fired and rehired multiple times, but the truth is that I just always managed to stay in the light.

One crazy event was when Greg Gaylord and I ran a transfer to Stanford in Palo Alto, and stopped for lunch at an old-school pizza place. We ordered a beer with our lunch, and since it tasted good, we decided to have another. There is no law against drinking a beer with a meal while on duty, as long as you don't drive under the influence. Craig Riggs, on more than one occasion, would show up and buy us a lunch that included alcohol. After lunch, we decided that the best way back to Merced was to grab Hwy 17 through Santa Cruz and back over Hwy 152 through Pacheco Pass and into Los Banos. The radios were making a lot of noise, ruining our state mind, so they got turned down, down, down. Santa Cruz was beautiful, so we stopped for a quiet walk on the beach. When we arrived back in Merced, and realized we were not hearing any radio traffic, we turned up our unit's radio and they were asking for us to report to the office. A three-hour return trip took six hours. I said, "Sorry we got lost, and no we did not hear you calling us on the radio."

I had the highest rate of non-transports and was always a leader in the complaint department. I once received three complaints in one day. The dispatcher, Gary Price, called me up laughing when he told me that the first complaint was for causing an indentation in the sheetrock of an obese patient's mobile home when we were returning him to his residence. The second complaint was for refusing to transport an elderly lady seeking pain medication, and the third was for a cardiac arrest patient where the family accused us of taking the patients wedding ring and replacing it with a fake, exact replica. The third complaint made the other two seem insignificant and all were forgotten. I had no hard feelings for being terminated, and I was working for Turlock Ambulance Service the next week (and with a raise).

Back in Turlock, I was partnered up with Big John. Appropriately named as he weighed in at over three hundred pounds, John would always show up for work early and get things prepared for his shift while the previous shift was still in service. We would find him at the hospital as we came out from a run, in the back of the unit restocking and checking oxygen levels. John would tell my other partner, "Hey if you want to go home, you can. I won't put in for the hours. Just top it off with fuel on your way in and I will meet you there." On many other occasions, Big John would show up at a medical aid and send my other partner home in his truck. John appreciated working with me since I was the one who helped him get his position as an EMT for Turlock.

He always had the most meticulous uniform, highly polished boots, and, of course, the latest Blockbuster releases to watch in crew's quarters. John even brought logs and would build a fire in the fireplace during the winter.

One evening, we were dispatched to a transfer from Emanuel Medical Center ICU in Turlock to Memorial North Hospital in Modesto. When we arrived at the hospital for the pickup and rolled our gurney down the hallways and into ICU, we found that our patient was in excess of 600 lbs. and was not going to fit on the gurney. We decided that we would leave our gurney there and attempt to slide the patient, mattress and all into the ambulance. As I was getting report from one nurse, another nurse who was going to ride with us to assist ventilations told me, "Be careful of that tube." I knew that she was referring to the endotracheal tube, but I replied, "What tube?" The nurse pointed to the ET tube coming out of the patient's mouth, to which the ventilator was hooked up. She told me for a third time that whatever I do, do not touch that tube. She said none of the hospital physicians could intubate the patient, and they had to have a two separate anesthesiologists come and perform the procedure. After wheeling the patient down the hallways to the ambulance bay, we matched the hospital bed as best as possible to the floor of the unit and with eight people all helping, we managed to get the leviathan loaded.

Celeste, the R.N. who was riding with us, is up in the front jump seat assisting ventilations. Being the jerk I can sometimes be and not able to get over being told not to touch the tube, I tease her by asking if she has brought her credit card. Celeste asks why, and I promptly tell her that on the way back from the transfer we are stopping for dinner and it is tradition for the rider to buy. She replies "Oh, I did not know we were stopping for dinner." After reaching Memorial North Hospital, unloading the behemoth of a patient, and transferring patient care, we started the return trip back to Turlock with our nurse and no gurney. About halfway back, in Ceres on South bound Hwy 99, we heard the other Turlock Ambulance, who was on the scene of a big rig vs. car, calling for back up. We were the closest ambulance, and those were our co-workers and friends calling for help. Big John stomped down on the accelerator and put us en-route. The wreck was out on Santa Fe, just South of Ballico. It was a twenty-minute drive that John managed to cut down to fifteen. As we pulled up, we saw over 100 feet of flares laid out on the road with three fire trucks and two CHP cars all with lights flashing. A semi-truck with two trailers was on its side with almonds spread all over the roadway. I stepped out to see my friend Erick, a new paramedic that I had trained, climbing out of a smashed, rolled-over car. Eric told me that there were two patients: one trapped in the car for whom he had called Medi-Flight, and a female that he found self-extricated and walking around upon his arrival. Eric stated to me that the female had been placed on a back board with a c-collar, was fully immobilized, and ready to go. We did not have a gurney, so we loaded the patient onto the bench seat in the back of the rig, where the nurse was waiting with her jaw dropped, asking what she could do. I asked her to get a blood pressure while I did a primary exam, and placed the patient on oxygen and the EKG monitor. The female patient was alert and oriented and while she had been involved in a serious collision and rollover, had no complaints. We started the ride to Emanuel ER and as I finished my secondary survey, I noticed that her abdomen was somewhat firm to palpation. Celeste told me her blood pressure is 130/82 with a heart rate of 98 and respirations of 16 a minute. I set up an IV bag of Normal Saline, tore some tape and grabbed a 16ga catheter. After applying a tourniquet, I slid it into her right ac and tape it down. The monitor was now showing a heart rate of 120 bpm (beats per minute) and as I rechecked her blood pressure, I found it to be 92/60. I did not feel any broken ribs, but that did not mean that she might not have one. It's possible that one may have ruptured her spleen or caused some other type of internal bleeding. I opened up the IV and administered a 500cc fluid bolus. The second IV that I started was, again, Normal Saline, and I got a 14ga in the patients left arm. Another blood pressure is repeated with a reading of 84/60 with an increasing pulse rate of 140 bpm. The female patient was now starting to speak in repetitive sentences, wanting to know where she was and what happened. I called the base hospital and gave them a full med-net report as well as ETA. The patient had now become unresponsive to verbal questions and barely moved towards painful stimuli. I did not notice any maxillofacial trauma and as she was still breathing. Since an oral intubation would have been difficult in this position, I opted to nasally intubate her with a 7.0 endotracheal tube, which went in successfully. I secured the tube with cloth tape and hooked up an Ambu-bag to the oxygen. I asked Celeste to assist ventilations. We arrived at the hospital and gave patient report to the ER staff and physician. I looked over at Celeste and said, "By the way, that was a nasal intubation. Only physicians or paramedics are allowed to do that." She was very humble and stated that she had never witnessed anything like that before. I thanked her for her help, and then she stated, "I didn't do anything." I said, "Hey, believe it or not, just staying out of the way and offering your help was more than you can imagine. I would be totally lost in your ICU. It would be great if you come and ride with us sometime and let me buy you dinner." Celeste become a good friend since that ride and now always brags about paramedics.

I had just recently gone through my second divorce and bought my ex-wife, Chris's, portion of equity out of the new house we had purchased. Messing up my marriage with Chris was one of my biggest mistakes, although I did not realize it until years later. I moved in, and then rented the two vacant rooms to two other divorced paramedics; and the wild times began. Bucky had the first room, Scott the second, and I was in the master. I could pretty much successfully flirt with and get most any girl I wanted. Bucky, on the other hand, with his long curly blonde locks and piercing blue eyes, had the girls flirting with him. We used to call girls and ask them to come over and bring alcohol. We thought that was the best thing: having them drive to us *and* bring the alcohol. Steve would plug in his base guitar, crank up Garth Brooks on the high-end stereo system we had, and play along. The girls loved it, and soon Steve would have them in the kitchen area on the hardwood floor, teaching them line dances. We never really had any problems, aside from occasionally having to sort out a temper tantrum. This mostly happened when other girls would show up, unannounced, and run into their friends who were hanging out with us. I guess it is not a good idea to show up to bachelor pad without arrangements first. Bucky and I also went through a cowboy faze in which we would only wear wranglers, cowboy shirts, Baily cowboy hats, and Justin Roper boots. We had a fireman friend that had a ranch and several horses. We would go out riding and then practice roping for hours.

My first patient shooting had come while I was an intern on the ambulance, working third person for Mobile Life Support in Modesto. We were stationed at McHenery and Briggsmore at the McHenery mall, where, in the back, we had small crew's quarters that we shared with Doctors Ambulance. The two ambulance companies that covered Modesto at the time were Mobile Life Support and Doctors Ambulance, and the ambulances would rotate 911 calls. When the call came in for a shooting at Daily's Restaurant and Lounge, we were just across the street. There were no stand back orders in those days, so we drove right into the mayhem. There was a well-dressed female lying supine on the pavement with a small pool of blood on the blacktop next to her chest. We went to her first and found she was not breathing and did not have a pulse. I grabbed an Ambu-bag and was getting ready to start CPR when the fire department arrived. We heard two loud gun shots go off inside the lounge area. The police department showed up in a group of three cruisers, while a man ran outside the front doors of the establishment. One of the officers got out of his vehicle, gun drawn and preceded towards us, we had started CPR and the fire department had just joined in. As the officer approached us cautiously, I noticed the man who had run out of lounge was now running towards the officer's open patrol car door. I shouted to the officer and pointed. He, in turn, shouted "Freeze, hands in the air! Now or I will shoot you!" Other policeman surrounded the man with his arms now in the air, and took him down. My instructor, after seeing that the officers had gone into the building, told me to go and see if anyone else was shot. When I arrived inside, it was pure pandemonium. There were at least 100 restaurant and bar patrons in total chaos, but I only found one patient with a bullet wound in his right upper arm. I made a quick sling by unbuttoning his shirt and pulling up the right side under his elbow. I then fastened one button to the higher button hole on his shirt. Another ambulance came and took the patient, who was shot in the arm, to the hospital. I went back to help my instructor as the female traumatic arrest patient was being loaded up. Unfortunately, even with as close as we were to the shooting, and then being only a few blocks to the trauma center, the effort of resuscitation was in vain, as most traumatic cardiac arrests tend to be.

I was working Turlock Ambulance when I received my first officer-involved shooting. The Officer had pulled over a vagrant on a bicycle, just off of West Main and Soderqusit, at a small park. While he was talking with the suspect, he was suddenly lunged at and stabbed in the chest several times. Jim drew his standard issue Smith and Wesson 9mm and unloaded it, striking the victim multiple times. When we arrived in the Turlock unit, the whole area was taped off and every officer available was there. We pronounced the victim dead before we even got out of the ambulance and went quickly to check on the officer. He was badly shaken up and not very talkative, but his bullet-proof vest protected him from the knife attack and he wasn't hurt physically. The officer refused transport, so we walked over and checked the victim, who was clearly dead.

Chapter 7

Little Brother was my partner once again, since he had now joined forces with Turlock Ambulance Service. We have gained a little more experience as the years have rolled by. My favorite calls were in-house medical aids, and while I did enjoy single patient trauma, multiple patient trauma was always tough for me, so I suffered through it the best I could. With multiple patients, triage comes into play and I have to do the most good for the most patients. This means I cannot give one-on-one treatment, and I must organize and utilize available resources. This can be tough, as I often have to walk away from a critical patient and instruct others on what to do. In-house medical aids are less chaotic, and I can focus on my patient. My favorite calls are generally anything out of the norm that makes me scratch my head and dig deep.

It is lunchtime while on duty in Turlock which generally means taco truck for me. I am told that Turlock has the highest number of churches, Mexican restaurants, and taco trucks per capita in the state. Mexican food is my mainstay it is an art to have just the right amount of grease dripping from a taco, as it is having just the right amount of chili sauce. Brian and I headed to our favorite taco truck, where the owners see us regularly and appreciate our business. Brian has always bragged that I am the only paramedic he knows who can eat four tacos en-route to a code 3 call and be finished when we got there. Not much of a feat, really, since they are so good and won't taste the same in an hour. So, you wolf them down, along with a few jalapenos, and life is great. Early the next morning, before we arose from sleep, the tones went off loudly through the crew's quarters and up we went. I hurried to the restroom while Brian lite a Marlboro on his way to start up the ambulance. Dispatch told us we were responding to a forty year-old male who was unresponsive at 1510 Laurel Street. We arrived on-scene and walked into the small dilapidated home to find an elderly black woman sitting on the couch. I said, "Hello, what seems to be the problem?" "It's my son, he won't wake up" she pointed to the couch behind us where we noticed the forty year-old laying on his back, and in the dimness of the room, he certainly appeared to be dead. As I approached him, I noticed an occasional respiration, so I grabbed his wrist to check for a pulse. I was not feeling one and I noticed he was very cold. Well, he was breathing about six times a minute, so I thought to myself that while you can have a pulse and not be breathing, you can't breathe without a pulse. Little Brother grabbed an OPA and hooked up an Ambu-bag to our portable oxygen tank. He then asked, as he began to ventilate, if I wanted fire to respond. I told him to continue assisting ventilations and let's wait a minute on the fire department. I asked the elderly woman, who is extremely calm, what kind of medical history her son has and she replied "He just got out of drug rehabilitation and went out last night. This is the first I have seen of him this morning." I had Brian check his pupils and he said they were pin point, I drew up 2mg of Naloxone into a 3cc syringe and administered it IM. In about three minutes, the patient's respirations increased to 18 per minute. Thinking the problem was solved, I tried talking to the patient who still did not respond. I applied a sternal rub that increased until he moved both arms toward me. Brain had stopped assisting ventilations and was now getting a blood pressure. Brian is better than the machine with his blood pressures and he is always correct. Little Brother announces that the blood pressure is 98/64 and a pulse rate of 92. He next hooked up the EKG which showed normal sinus rhythm. I next asked the mother if she knew of any other medical problems her son may have and she stated no. I asked her to find all his medications for me as Brian set up an IV bag of Normal Saline and prepared the glucometer. The lady came back with several medications. One was Glyburide, a hypoglycemic medication for diabetics. Checking the patient's blood glucose with a drop of blood gave us a low reading, which meant it was generally below 20 micrograms per kilogram. I managed to start an 18ga angio catheter after two tough misses, and Brian hooked up the IV tubing and taped it in place while I retrieved the D-50. I pushed the 25g of D-50 while we loaded the patient onto the gurney and headed to the ambulance. We asked the mother if she would like to come with us, and she said she would get a ride in with a friend. Once in the back of the unit, I tried talking to the patient again but there was still no verbal response. I rechecked the patient's glucose level and it was now 52, which is still too low since 70-100 was normal. Brian jumped up front to drive and asked if I wanted code 3, I replied, "Not for now. Let me get another round of Dextrose in first." The second dose of D-50 brings the patient's blood glucose up to 140 mcg/kg and still no verbal response. I scratched my head and suddenly realized that the patient was still very cold. I turned up the heater and placed three blankets on and around the patient, along with two heat packs under his arm pits. I told Brian to pick it up to code 3, and I took a second set of vitals. His blood pressure was now 105/70 with a heart rate of 82 and respirations remained at 18. Time to radio the hospital. "Emanuel Medical Center, Emanuel Medical Center, Medic 201 on med channel five." "This is Emanuel the time is 0630 MICN Moeller go ahead please." "Good morning Emanuel this is

Turlock Medic 201 paramedic Coakley and EMT Sawyer en-route to your facility Code 3 with an ETA of approximately six minutes. We have a forty year-old male patient, approximately eighty kilograms onboard, who we were told was unresponsive. Upon our arrival, we found the patient to be non-verbal with an initial blood pressure of 98/64, pulse rate of 92 per minute, and respirations of 6- 8 per minute. We initially assisted respirations and after assessing his pupils found them to be pin point so we have administered 2mg of Naloxone IM. The patient's respirations increased to 18 per minute. Be advised we also discovered that the patient takes Glyburide and his glucose came back as low. We have given a total of two amps of Dextrose at 50% and have current blood glucose of 180 mcg/kg, a current blood pressure of 105/72, and pulse rate of 92. Corresponding with the monitor in normal sinus rhythm, the patient remains non-verbal. However, he does respond appropriately to painful stimuli. The patient is very cold to the touch, so we have the heater on, multiple blankets on him, and two hot packs under each arm pit. At this point we are thinking that the patient is hypothermic." "Copy Medic 201 we will see you inside, room 2 please." After arriving and transferring patient care, we resupplied the bus for the next call. Before leaving the hospital, we were told the patient was in fact hypothermic with a core temperature of just 88 degrees Fahrenheit.

Now that I was in Turlock, I was training paramedic students more often and my only prerequisite was that the student either be from Stanislaus County or was going to be working in the county. I did not believe in training the multitude of students who were flooding into the area to be trained, but then plan to work elsewhere. Paramedic field trainers were just creating competition for themselves if they decided to test for a fire department job outside of county. It had always been my philosophy to give back what was given to me, and teaching helped me do that. Some Field Training Officers (FTO's) did it for the extra pay or because they were lazy. They saw it as a way out of doing their job. They had the student wash, check out, and stock the ambulance, as well as do all the lifting and paperwork. In Turlock, we formed what we called "The Breakfast Club." We would meet up with the on-duty crews and off-going crews for breakfast at the Almond Tree (who fed us for half off), and we would grill the paramedic students with scenarios. The students would get so nervous sitting at a table with three or four paramedics (and another two or three EMT's) that they would start sweating. This was not about hazing in any way. It was about learning, for all of us. We would start off easy and work our way up. One of our paramedics, Bob Easter, would never let a student save a patient. He always devised his scenarios to go any direction the student picked, but would always toss in a curve ball at the end. One such example would be to start the student on a chest pain scenario and tell them any information they wanted; they just had to ask.

"You respond code 3 to a 55 year old male who is complaining of chest pain. Take it from there."
"Ok, I ask the patient when the pain started and what it feels like."
"The pain started about 20 minutes ago and feels like a heavy pressure. Next?"
"I have the patient placed on oxygen at 6 liters per nasal cannula."
"Ok"
"I place the patient on the EKG monitor. What do I see?"
"Ventricular tachycardia."
"Do I have a blood pressure?"

"Do you?"

"Ok, I take a blood pressure, and...?"

"72/42. Do you know why?"

"No"

"Because the patient has been in ventricular tachycardia since you arrived. Do you know what you could have done differently?"

"I should have made patient contact by introducing myself and feeling for a radial pulse. That way I would have known if his skin was cool or clammy verses warm and hot and, most importantly, if a radial pulse was present and was strong, weak, or irregular."

"Good"

"Ok, I give Lidocaine. Correction, I cardiovert the patient."

"Ok, what setting?"

"100 joules."

"Ok, the patient converts to normal sinus with a heart rate of 80 and blood pressure of 150/90"

"Alright, I want to know the patients past medical history and has this ever happened before. I want an IV of D-5W with an 18ga angio catheter, make that a liter of Normal Saline, instead."

"Ok, this has not happened before, and the patient has a past medical history of hypertension and hyperlipidemia."

"Alright, I administer .4mg of nitroglycerin sublingual, any changes?"

"The patient says that he feels dizzy and the alarm on the monitor goes off. You look and see a run of 6 premature ventricular contractions."

"Ok, I administer 100mg of Lidocaine, are we at the hospital yet?"

"No, your patient is now having seizure activity."

"Ok, I administer 4mg of Valium. Any change?"

"No"

"I call the base and give a med-net; are we almost there?"

"Two minutes"

"Ok, I administer my second dose of Valium 2mg IVP."

"Ok, you arrive at the emergency room with the patient still seizing. The doctor and family are in the room and the doctor asks how much Lidocaine you have administered to patient, since the patient has seizures if given Lidocaine." The five patient's rights are 1. Right patient 2. Right dose 3. Right drug 4. Right route 5. Right date.

Chapter 8

The weather was warming up, and the wild times at the home for wayward paramedics were in full swing. Steve was dating an old flame named Andrea, and I was dating Lisa and Jennifer, and Jenifer and Lisa, it was like this and like that most of the summer to come. Bucky and Andrea were now on again, off again, and Steve moved on to Jill, a CDF firefighter he met while working in "Hooterville". We took Jill and Jenifer to Shore Line for a Travis Tritt concert, and we rented one room at the Hyatt Hotel with two queen sized beds. We filled the sink in the front of the bathroom with ice and cans of Coors Light, bottles of Zima, and two bottles of Crown Royale with a stack of red Solo cups sit on the counter. Luckily for us, both girls had just turned twenty-one, so the alcohol was not a legal problem. The morning of the concert, we loaded our ice chest with our beer and poured the Crown into two flasks. Since they don't allow bottles, the Zima stayed in the hotel. I called for the prearranged limousine service to pick us up out front, and when we arrived at the concert, we made our way through the crowds to find a spot to sit on the grassy hill that overlooks the stage. Travis did not let us down. He rolled out on a Harley and performed an absolutely awesome concert. Bucky and I, like the girls, were dressed in Wranglers and Justin Roper boots (and, of course, Baily straw cowboy hats). Leaving the concert, we had both of the girls on our shoulders and we walked side by side, carrying the large the ice chest between us when I stepped into a gopher hole and went down, ass over tea kettle. Luckily not hurting Jennifer, who went down with me. My ankle twisted and dislocated, and then relocated itself. The swelling was unbelievable, and after returning to the room and finally getting my boots off. I limped and wore a brace for over a year after that. Of course, I never sought medical attention.

Back at work in Turlock, I was working with Rob Lyons, and we discussed a call years earlier, while I was training with Alan Kissling. He was one of my field training officers and another paramedic who was certified in the 70's. Alan did three tours in Vietnam as a Ranger receiving two Silver Stars, one Bronze Star, and the Purple Heart. Kissling was built like Pappy Boyington, and he would have occasional mood swings that would make even a lion cower. I saw him grab a doctor by his jacket, and pull him over to the patient whom we were transporting from Emanuel Medical Center, to a nursing home across the street. "Do you see this? This patient should not be discharged, the patient is going to expire at any moment and the nursing staff across the street will be calling us right back." The reply from the physician was just a mumble of "sorry" and "This is not my patient", as he scampered away. When riding third person with Alan as my instructor, we were dispatched to a motor vehicle accident in Hilmar on August road. When we pulled on-scene, there were two cars that were in a head-on collision at high speed. Young teenage bodies were scattered over the ground, not moving and never to move again. There were a total of seven teenagers, five of whom we declared dead at the scene, and two whom were prepared for transport. The first patient, who was c-collared and immobilized on a back board, stopped breathing as we loaded him in. He still had a faint pulse as I grabbed the Ambu-bag and started ventilating while Alan set up for an intubation attempt. Alan, unable to intubate because of the severe facial trauma, quickly performed a cricothyroid needle insufflation with a 12ga Angio-catheter. I was watching over his shoulder when he barked at me to get vitals on the second patient, "Do something for someone we can help."

After arriving at the hospital and patient number one being declared dead, patient two was x-rayed and checked over, but somehow he had no significant injuries. We learned that the kids who were sophomores, were on lunch break and playing chicken. I don't think there was a winner of that game; it was always tragic when youth meet sudden death.

Turlock Ambulance had a competitive softball team for decades, and it was a great way to interact with the public, as well the police department, who also made up part of our team. One night while on duty, the team was short one player, so my partner Rob Lyons and I rolled down to the ball park and I suited up in my elastic shorts, knee brace, and team shirt. After hitting a double and standing on second base, a medical aid was dispatched to us. It was for a seventy-two year-old female with a fall and left hip pain. We had to call a time out as I sprinted off the field towards the ambulance, it was hot out and I was sweating, so I decided to run the medical aid in my softball uniform. The firemen thought it was funnier than hell, and the patient was happy with my treatment. However upon arrival to the hospital, several nurses complained because I didn't take the patient to the hospital where she had medical coverage. They thought I was just trying to dump the patient on them so I could get back to playing softball. While that may or may not be true, my job is to simply transport patients to the closet hospital that can treat their specific problem. In this case, the patient had an apparent left hip fracture and we were closest to Turlock, the patients insurance coverage was supposedly for Memorial Medical Center in Modesto. It is not my responsibility as a paramedic to ask for or verify insurance information prior to hospital transport. To do so would be against my oath as a paramedic by making insurance or non-insurance destination decisions. Having been in the ambulance business as an owner of Valley Springs Ambulance Service, I was aware that insurance companies would pay for the ambulance and hospital services in an emergency situation, and may in fact charge the patient for a longer transport destination. The rub here is that most of the large ambulance providers want the hospitals happy, and of course the patients as well. So they put pressure on the transporting units to take patients where ever they wanted to go. The problem with this is that while transporting a patient with a serious medical problem, such as shortness of breath, and the patients preferred hospital is 20 miles further than the closest facility, things can and will go wrong. This leaves the transporting team in a possible situation for litigation and more importantly the possibility of losing a patient. Of course in this case, a fractured left hip is generally stable, and it is more of a patient comfort situation. Bouncing down the road any further than need be, in my opinion was not the best solution. I would simply explain the situation to the patient, and they would most often agree. Of course once at the local hospital, the overloaded staff is not encouraging any more patients then possible.

Two exceptions to the rule are major trauma related cases that fit in a special triage category, they require transport past a possible closer facility that is not a designated a receiving Level 2 Facility. The Level 2 Trauma Facilities are required to have a full and ready operating room, and team immobilized within 20 minutes, ready for immediate surgery. The time starts when the paramedic calls in before and or while transporting. The second rule is patients in the process of an acute mi (myocardial infarction, heart attack) as confirmed by a 12 lead EKG, and the paramedic, as having ST(the ST is a segment of the EKG) elevation in two or more leads. This has been found to be 95 percent accurate in all chest pain patients. These candidates go to the closest approved STEMI Center, where again the facility and team must be ready and waiting the paramedics team arrival. These have both been major changes made in the last several years.

The 72-hour work week had dropped to a 60-hour work week with the same pay. I now came in Sunday night at 6 p.m. and work until Wednesday morning at 6 a.m. This gave me 4 ½ days off each week, I just needed to power through a 2 ½day shift. We had just finished some great burritos from Sylvester's Viva La Taco bus when our radios and pagers sounded, "Medic 201 respond code 3 for a fainting at the Holy Cross Church in the back conference room," "10-4," replied Brian as he raced out of the crews quarters ahead of me to light his usual cigarette. He inhaled three puffs before stomping it out. Sometimes I would go slowly to let Brian get an extra puff, and other times I would move more quickly to stop him from having a chance to light up; it depended upon whether or not he was talking about quitting. We arrived at the medical aid, pulled our gurney out of the ambulance, and began walking towards the back of the church when we were flagged over to the conference room. We stepped into the conference room where there was about twenty people seated at two long tables with their bibles opened. The patient was in her 60s and was lying on her back with a pillow under her head, her knees up, and a man by her side. I asked what happened as I got on one knee and took the patients wrist, feeling a regular pulse. The man said he was a doctor and that the patient passed out while sitting at the table. I asked if she struck her head when she hit the floor and I was told no, she passed out and was laid on the ground. Noticing that the patient had vomited, I asked her if she vomited before passing out or after. The patient, who was alert, answered that she vomited afterwards. I asked if this had happened before and she stated, no. I asked "What kind of medical problems do you have?" She answered that she was a diabetic and confirmed she had recently eaten. The doctor, who was getting annoyed at my questions, told me that he was her physician. I replied, "What are the chances of that? It's good that you happened to be here." Brian placed the patient on oxygen and was getting vitals, with that done he then looked up at me. I pointed to my chest and then the monitor indicating to place the patient on the EKG machine. The doctor interrupted: "That won't be necessary. I have already called the hospital and arranged for her to be admitted to the floor." Trying to be polite, which is not always in my nature when I am focused on the job at hand, I asked if he would like us to start an IV. He replied, "No." I asked "Ok, would you like us to get a glucose reading on the way over," he replied "That's fine; just get moving. They are expecting her." he replied. We loaded up the patient, while I continuously asked the patient medical questions. "Do you have any chest pain? Did you feel dizzy or your heart racing before passing out?" She stated no to both questions and claimed she just blacked out. As we were rolling her outside on the gurney, I asked Brian why he did not place the patient on the monitor. He responded, "The doctor said not to." I replied, "I don't care what the doctor said, when I ask you to do something, you do it." He repeated, "I know, but the doctor said not to." When we loaded the patient in the back of the ambulance, I asked Brian to put the patient on the monitor, which he did while looking at me like I was losing it. With the EKG monitor attached, Little Brother runs a strip and handed it to me, looking at the strip I identified an obvious ST elevation which is indicative of a myocardial infarction, or in other words, a significant heart attack that was presently happening. I asked Brian to hang me a line of Normal Saline and tear some tape. He was in the game now and understood my concern. This was our patient and the outcome was up to us, whether or not a doctor was on-scene. I started the IV in the left hand with an 18ga angio catheter and taped it down. Brian placed a drop of blood on the glucometer, which gave us a normal reading of 88mkg/kg. Our current vital signs were, blood pressure: 168/88, pulse rate: 88 and respirations of 18. Most people have chest pain when they are having a heart attack and usually (but not always) pain down the left arm. Diabetics, however, often have no signs at all. We started for Emanuel ER and I administered the patient .4mg of Nitroglycerin under her tongue, followed by 324 mg of aspirin. I then contacted the hospital on the med net radio and gave them a full report. I included that the patient's physician was on-scene, and had arranged for her to be a direct admit, however we have found the patient to have ST elevation. "Copy, Medic 201 we will see you inside" When we rolled inside and attempted to go into the emergency room, we are stopped by the charge nurse who asked if that was the direct admit. I stated "Yes, but she has ST elevation and should be seen here." The nurse replied that they are waiting for her upstairs. I replied, "O.K., as long as you understand that I believe she is infracting right now." We started down the hall when the nursing supervisor, Benny Diaz, asked me what was going on. I explained quickly as we rolled down the hallway and into the elevator. When we reached the patient's room, and before we could unload her, Benny asked me, "Do you think she is having an MI?" "Yes", I replied. Benny stated, "They don't even have telemetry on this floor; hold on." Benny called ICU to get a room available for the patient and a team prepared for an MI in progress. "Bill, I am so sorry. Can you take her to the ICU for me?" "Of course, thank you so much. I am glad you were there." When we entered into the ICU, a team of six members was waiting to accept the patient and report. After moving the patient over to her bed and giving a patient report, we went about remaking the gurney with sheets from the ICU and putting our EKG cables back together and into the monitor case. The ICU team had finished a 12 lead EKG and confirmed that the patient was, in fact, infracting. They then prepared a Streptokinase drip, which is an anti-thrombolytic agent, used to dissolve vascular clots.

Brian stopped in the ER on the way back to our unit to wash his hands, and the ER doctor (who was yawning and taking a pretend golf swing) asked if the patient had indigestion? Brian said, "No, an MI. They are putting her on a Streptokinase drip in the ICU." Outside the ER we are putting the gurney into the ambulance, when Brian said "I know I screwed up." "Good enough for me, buddy. We are responsible for the patient unless the doctor wants to come along and, in this case, I was not going to ask. I felt it would be better for the patient if we did it our way."

A week later, we heard a nurse saying to the ER doctor, "Well the paramedics should have just brought the patient into the ER anyways that's their job"

Off-duty for four days and I was dating a gal by the name of Michele whom I met while shopping at the Big 5 sporting goods store in Turlock. She was majoring in criminal science at Stanislaus State University. Her brother played Triple-A ball for the Dodgers, and her father was the Northern territory distributor for Ram golf clubs. Her mother had remarried an attorney, and lived in Discovery Bay, on the golf course. Michele and I were headed out to Monterey to do some scuba diving and just hang out. We thought maybe we'd catch some jazz at one of the many pubs that had live music that night. We arrived at our motel that catered to scuba divers. They had large barrels of water to clean your wet suits and gear, which was better than having to bring them into the shower and get sand everywhere. We stopped by one of the local dive shops to inquire about the conditions (like visibility), and found that Break Water had the best current conditions. I had been scuba diving since 1975 which was the year Jaws came out. While not a very physical sport, it is always an adventure. That night, we went out for dinner on the pier and walked around until we found a small bar that had some live jazz. Michele was wearing a backless black dress and pumps, and I was wearing blue jeans with a t-shirt and flip flops. We had several drinks, so we decided to leave my truck and walk back to the motel. When we reached the motel, Michele took off running ahead of me. I took off after her, picking up her pumps, black nylons, and lastly her dress at the doorway to the room. I entered the room where she was waiting in bed. Wow, women are good. We flew to Mexico for one vacation and hung out with her family, and on another went to her folk's beach house in Parajo Dunes. Right when I was beginning to think she was pretty special, she proved me wrong. We had dated almost a year when I noticed she was not answering my calls. She had started dating a sheriff and, instead of telling me, she left me to figure it out on my own—not cool. Of course she tried to come back about six months later, but I like to move forward and not backward. I had finally learned that a serious relationship takes honesty, trust, and monogamy to last. I had caused more than my fair share of heartache, so it was my turn to get a taste of it myself.

Chapter 9

Once again, back in Turlock I was fast asleep and halfway thru my 60-hour shift when the tones went off. I awoke, startled, not knowing where I was. I felt my chest getting tight and my pulse starting to race as I opened my eyes into darkness. "Medic 201, respond code 3 to 1808 Sunbird St. for an 80 year-old male; difficulty breathing." Rubbing my eyes as I rolled out of bed, the brunette named Theresa, who was lying next to me, never even flinched. I could hear Brian across the crew's quarters getting up and mumbling to himself. He probably couldn't find his cigarettes. The owner of Turlock Ambulance did not care if we had sleepovers as long as he never saw them. As Little Brother fired up the unit, we heard the fire department going en-route across town. The other Turlock ambulance was on a call, so we needed to make up some time and get to the call a little faster than usual since it was on the far side of town. When we got there and pulled out our gurney with all the needed equipment, we rolled into the hallway where we were greeted by a not-too-happy black female wanting to know what took us so long. "Sorry ma'am. It is busy out there tonight. Who are we here for?" "It's my father; he is in the back room. Hurry, this is a bunch of bullshit; if we were white, you would have already been here." We walked into the bedroom to find a friendly-looking man of eighty years, sitting up and leaning forward with his feet hanging off the side of the bed, gasping for breath. It did not take a rocket scientist to see the swelling in his ankles and hear the crackling of his breath; he was in CHF (congestive heart failure) and was deteriorating rapidly. The daughter was screaming at us to hurry up and get him to the hospital, and then yelling that he needed to go to Doctor's Medical Center in

Modesto. I looked at her father and then at her and I told her that he needs to go to the closest emergency room otherwise he might not make it. She started screaming at us again, so I asked the firemen to calm her down and keep her away from us. Brian had the patient on high-flow oxygen by mask and advised me that the blood pressure was 210/160. "Ok, let's put him on the monitor and get to the unit." The patient was in a sinus tachycardia at 130 bpm with respirations of 40 per minute. The pulse oximetry was 78% when we loaded him into the unit. Inside the ambulance, Brian scrambled to set up an IV of Normal Saline while I administered Nitroglycerin 1.2mg sublingual, which were three sprays under the tongue. Placing a tourniquet around the patients left arm and fruitlessly searched for a vein. I grabbed the patients hand and vigorously slapped the top of it; still nothing. I reached for the Nitroglycerin, sprayed one squirt to the top of the patient's left hand, and a vein began to puff out. Luckily, I managed to place an 18ga angio catheter in the left hand and taped it in place. I set the IV at TKO (to keep open) and continued reassessing the patient, who was not getting any better. The patient was getting tired and increasingly diaphoretic. I looked at the monitor, and his heart rate was slowing down to 60 bpm "Little Brother do you see that?" Brian knew what I had in mind as I reached for the intubation kit and he answered, "It looks like a possible seizure." "Yes, probably hypoxic, draw me 10mg of valium" Unfortunately, we did not have RSI (rapid sequence intubation) in our protocols. This allows you to sedate and paralyze the patient so you can take over their breathing. In the future there will be CPAP (continuous positive airway pressure), but at this time it was not available. I could try a nasal intubation, however with the patient leaning forward, in a tri-pod position with his head down, this would be difficult for both myself and the patient. It has been impossible at any point to assist ventilations with the Ambu-bag as the patient is leaning forward. I pushed the valium and counted to ten, laid the patient flat, and Brian started to ventilate. I inserted the laryngoscope blade under the patients tongue and lifted while Brian pushed on the patient's trachea. I watched the vocal cords come into view and slide the 8.0 ET past them as they opened. I took over assisting ventilations with one hand and fumbled for Lasix, which is a diuretic, with the other. I drew up 80 mg, which is double the amount our patient took on a daily basis. I then asked Brian, "How about a nice, easy code 3 to Emanuel?" Brain has already jumped out of the back and is now in the front, about to take off, when the patient's daughter starts hitting the side of the ambulance with her fists. She is cussing at us to give her father back to her. I locked the back doors and we drove to the hospital, the patient's daughter followed us through red lights the entire way. I called report to the hospital on the med-net radio, while Brian had contacted dispatch, requesting that the police department meet us at Emanuel, he also requested dispatch to advise Emanuel Security to be waiting for us in the ambulance bay. Upon arrival at the hospital, we unloaded the patient, who was looking much better now. The daughter arrived on our heels only to be intercepted by security and was ranting and raving like crazy. We exchanged patient care with the ER and gave a full detailed report to the staff and attending physician.

The patient's daughter was in room 7, with the police department detaining her, when Little Brother walked over for damage control. She was having nothing to do with Brian's attempt to apologize and explain the seriousness of her father's condition. Brian looked to the police officer who was getting tired of the daughter's attitude and the officer asked Brian if he wanted to press charges for interfering with an Advanced Life Support Unit? Little Brother looked at the lady and said he didn't think that would be beneficial. He just wanted her to understand that we were doing our best to keep her father alive. He stated that if she does not escalate the problem any further, he was willing to let it go. She agreed and, of course, a week later the complaint came in.

Chapter 10

When I first started working as a paramedic, I was hired by San Andres Ambulance and my first partner ever was Bob Easter. Bob was always paranoid and refused to talk to me if anyone else was around. He would always say, "Come here, come here." And while we talked, he would be looking around constantly. Bob had a way of making me feel like we were the Secret Service, surrounded by spies. Bob would drink coffee all day and night, and smoke cigarette after cigarette. Our very first call was a motor vehicle vs. big rig on Hwy 26 out of Valley Springs. Bob was driving code 3 like a bat out of hell, and was not talking while he focused on the road. It was almost lunch time, so I asked him what he felt like for lunch. He looked at me and said. "What?" I said "Can I buy you lunch if we are still alive after this call?" That's when we heard a loud boom from the engine and smoke started billowing into the cab. "Bob, call for backup", I shouted as I clambered into the back of the ambulance through the small cubby hole that separated the front from the back. I hooked up two oxygen masks and then slid back up front. "I have back up coming. I think we can make it; we are almost there", Bob said. We had both of our windows down and through the smoke, I could barely make Bob out as I handed him an oxygen mask. Up ahead I could see a vehicle that ran under the trailer of a big rig and was now sitting there looking like a custom-made convertible. When we stepped out of the ambulance with the engine knocking and smoke pouring out, the fire department was not sure if they were happy to see us or not. There were two patients: one walking around looking confused, and the other spitting up blood and teeth. Bob grabbed the suction and went right to work, I asked the fire department get the other patient, who was a twenty-five year-old female. They sat her down on a backboard while holding her neck and head in a neutral position and immobilized her. Bob was like a wizard doing multiple things at once, stuck on high speed. He had the fire department cutting off the clothes of patient number one, who was the driver and had been pulled out of the wreckage by bystanders. Bob was alternating oxygen and suction for the patient as needed. I had firemen getting vitals on patient number two while I did a secondary exam on both patients. The first patient appeared to have fractured jaw and a broken upper left arm; however his chest and abdomen seemed fine, which was most important. Patient number two had an obvious concussion, but was otherwise checking out well. The driver of the big rig denied treatment and told us he had just pulled out onto the road when the car came speeding at him. *We will let CHP figure that one out,* I thought to myself. I went for the unit's radio to check on our back up and see if a helicopter could meet us, since it was looking like this should be a transport to Stockton. The radio was working, but we were in dead spot. Let's hope our last transmission got through. Patient number one was doing better after Bob had suctioned his airway; he was fully immobilized, on a back board, with a c-collar in place and has a blood pressure of 122/70, a pulse of 78, and respirations of 16. Patient number two had a blood pressure of 118/77, a pulse of 88 and respirations of 18. The second ambulance arrived and had a paramedic on board named Dale. He was half owner of San Andreas Ambulance Service, along with his sister, Gail. Dale asked if we wanted to take the two patients on to Stockton in his ambulance or stay here and wait for the tow truck that was on its way. Before Bob could say "let's go to Stockton", I thanked Dale and told him we would stay there.

After starting as a paramedic with San Andrea's Ambulance in Calaveras County, the owners Dale and Gail Jones, decided to expand their operations and take over the other ambulance companies with their new paramedic service. They started by buying a four wheel drive ambulance and placing it up in Arnold. There were now three ambulance services rotating 911 calls in the small mountain town. The county did not differentiate Calaveras Ambulance's EMT 2 service or San Andrea's paramedic service, from Arnold Ambulance's EMT 1 service, so the 911 medical aids were rotated. The plan was to thin the herd by financially "knocking out" the other two providers. It probably would have worked if was not for Big Bill Macfall, who was an employee of Calaveras Ambulance. He was furious that they placed an ambulance in Arnold on the far South side of the county, but left Valley Springs to their Northeast to be covered by themselves from San Andreas. He gave the ultimatum that if San Andreas Ambulance did not pull out of Arnold, he would start an ambulance service in Valley Springs, where he lived and worked on the volunteer fire department. Bill waited three months to no avail and started up Valley Springs Ambulance Service with his wife Janis, who was an RN/paramedic.

All the calls in Valley Springs that used to get dispatched to San Andreas Ambulance were dispatched to Valley Springs Ambulance. San Andreas Ambulance responded by flexing its muscles and placed another unit in Valley Springs to cause a rotation of calls. Big Bills son-in-law was a paramedic and lived in San Andreas. He got into the fight by opening Professional Ambulance Service and based it in San Andreas, causing yet another rotation of 911 calls. Let the ambulance wars begin; it was getting crazy.

I was working in Valley Springs with Don Zyski as my EMT partner. He was 62 years-old with salt and pepper hair and a soft, likable smile. It was deer-hunting season, when we caught a call to Blue Mountain for a hunter who fell off a cliff and had broken his leg. As we went en-route, we heard the Ebbetts Pass Search and Rescue Team dispatched for the call. We traveled about forty-five minutes out into the country and finally down a dirt road to where the Sheriff's Department and Ebbetts Pass SAR (search and rescue) had set up a base camp. We got out of the rig, headed towards the base camp, and learned that the patient was approximately three miles in, stuck on the face of a cliff that he had fallen down. We then learned that Fallon Air Force Base had a Chinok rescue helicopter on its way to coordinate the evacuation. It was a beautiful afternoon with the sun low in the sky and scattered cumuliform clouds threatening a thunderstorm and some much-needed rain. We needed to get in and get the patient out before the evening set in. We grabbed back packs and loaded cardboard splints, tape, IV supplies, and a mixture of emergency medications, including Morphine and Demerol, for pain. The Ebbetts Pass Search and Rescue Team was equipped with climbing ropes, carabineers, and a Stokes Basket, as well as lights, water, and food supplies in case we did not complete our objective as planned. We started off down a steep trail, twelve of us in all. The SAR Team had communications with the base camp and was aware of our coordinates from a Sheriff's Department helicopter. They had made visual contact with the patient earlier. The route we followed was a small, dry, hard packed deer trail that we walked in single file. We hiked for what seemed like forever, climbing over fallen trees and through unforgiving brush that scratched at any uncovered surface on our bodies. We finally reached a precipice that was 100 feet above the patient, where his son was awaiting us. He told us that his father was looking over the cliff with his binoculars when he slipped and fell. Luckily they had a cell phone, and the son was able to contact the sheriff's office. The search and rescue team went to work belaying ropes to repel down to the victim. Fortunately I had taken several survival training courses, and had worked with Ebbetts Pass FD practicing repelling from their tower at the fire station. I slipped into my harness, and Captain Bill Becker and I descended slowly and safely to the patient's side without a problem. Bill radioed to send down two more members of the rescue team. I introduced myself and Bill to the patient, and reached for a pulse in his wrist while asking questions to ascertain his level of consciousness. I asked "Did you strike your head?" and "Where do you hurt?" the patient responded, "No, I did not hit my head but my right lower leg hurts like hell; I think it is broken." I did a quick head-to-toe exam and after cutting his trousers and examining his lower leg, I found he had an obviously deformed tibia and fibula. The rest of the exam revealed he was otherwise sound. His distal pulses to the injury were intact, so I grabbed a quick set of vitals and listened to his lungs; they sounded normal. I asked if he had any other medical problems or if he was allergic to any medication and he replied "no" to both questions. I then asked if he was opposed to some pain medication, since it was going to be bump and go to get him out of here. He said that would be great, so I drew 100 mg of Demerol and gave him an IM (intra muscular) shot in his left buttocks. The next two members of the SAR team made their way down with a Stokes Litter Basket. We splinted the obviously-fractured leg with cardboard and towels, and lifted the patient gently into the litter basket. Bill attached two ropes to the litter: one to pull the patient up, and the other as a safety line. Then we four clipped ourselves on to the basket with a short piece of rope and a carabineer. Bill also clipped a radio ear piece on and called up to have the team above initiate the pulling. We moved upwards in three-foot short pulls, clipped to the basket sometimes helping move it forward and other times, the basket was keeping us from tumbling back down the cliff. Once we made it to the top, we hiked another mile to a clearing where the Chinook from Fallon Air Force Base had an ETA of 15 minutes. While we waited, I set up a bag of Lactated Ringers and started a 16ga angio catheter in Curt's left arm. The Chinook, now overhead, lowers a cable and harness for the Stokes Litter Basket. SAR attaches it, and the patient is lifted aboard the helicopter.

Bob Easter and I were still working for San Andreas Ambulance in the Valley Springs unit, when the money got tight and Gail decided, that we could no longer leave the crew's quarters to eat or run an occasional errand. Gail being frustrated by the economic damage she had started, compromised her business again by taking it one step further and removing the crew's quarter's phone so we could no longer talk to our families. Almost a year of this craziness continued, until one day when Big Bill stopped by and offered to sell me his ambulance service. He wanted no money down, just take over and make payments on the equipment. I had a better idea. I talked to Bob Easter and we approached Bill with an idea to do a three-way partnership. One month later, Valley Springs Ambulance had two new partners and we were in on the ambulance wars.

When Bob and I became partners and owners of Valley Springs Ambulance, we were available on all our off days for Valley Springs, our new company. After five months, San Andreas Ambulance pulled out. Bob and I also worked for Sierra Construction, who was putting in a dam and water-diverting tunnels at Spicer Reservoir. It was a five year project, and I happened to fall into the position as their first paramedic. As such, they had me in charge of setting up ambulances and equipment for their remote sites. Cal Osha required medical services at all times when working was in progress. I was in charge of hiring nurses and paramedics, and of course, I put Bob on the job. The shifts were twelve hours, around the clock. One day, a dozer operator rolled off a cliff at my site. After calling for a helicopter, I responded to the victim and, with help from the construction workers, got him fully immobilized and c-collared with a full set of vitals and two large bore IVs prior to the helicopter landing. It was the only real excitement for the majority of the project, but the medical benefits were great and the pay was even better. Sierra Construction was a subsidiary of Guy F. Attkinson which, at the time, was the fourteenth largest construction company in the world. They built bridges and dams throughout the entire country and abroad. Bob and I also worked part-time on the ambulance in Merced. We would have about one day off work every three weeks, and it was crazy. Bob and I finally got burnt out from all the work so we sold out to our third partner and original owner Bill McFall.

Chapter 11

On another warm summer night with a full moon in the works, I was working Turlock Ambulance with Rich Murdock, (Mud was his softball nick name). We had Big John riding with us, since he had been bumped down to wheelchair service. Turlock Ambulance was starting to double up on paramedics, working two together to better utilize our workforce. Big John would cover any ALS (advanced life support) he could get and would ride along at night with Mud and myself. The tones went off and set us in motion for a reported 30 year-old male in cardiac arrest at the VFW (Veterans of Foreign Wars) hall on East Linwood. We arrived on-scene and walked in, loaded for bear with all of our equipment loaded on the gurney, only to find a 30 year-old male who was intoxicated and laying on his back. Rich got on one knee to talk to him, and the patient raised his right arm to swing at him, so I quickly fell forward with my right knee in his chest. Before I could stand up, a middle-aged man came running at me with both fists out. I managed to get up quickly, avoid his onslaught of swings, and push him backwards and he stumbled falling to the ground. I looked around the bar area and there were more than twenty pissed off people moving our way. I glanced behind me and could only see the back of Big John as he was swinging his massive arms and fists back and forth with bodies tumbling left and right. Mud calls for police backup and, before bad could get worse, Murdock stood up and yelled at the crowd, "Back up now. Every one of you not back against that wall is going to jail; the police are on their way."

When the Turlock Police Department arrived, it was a canine unit with Officer Finn Johnson. Finn asked me what happened and I briefly explained. He asked who was involved, so I replied, "that individual." I pointed to the middle-aged gentleman sitting at the bar who had tried to attack me. Finn instructed him, "Hands on your head now." He grabbed his handcuffs with one hand and pushed the perpetrators head down to the bar with the other. After he handcuffed him, he asked, "Ok, who else?" The three of us: Mud, Big John, and I pointed out the other two drunken VFW wannabe fight contenders. Finn and his canine partner loaded up all three and took them to jail; striking, or attempting to strike, a paramedic is a felony.

In the morning, we went to the Almond Tree for breakfast. I was training two students this year: Richard Sealander and Bob Vargas, both friends with each other, and both lived in Patterson. I would have Rich for a 24- hour shift, and then Bob for the next 24- hours. It was my turn to form a scenario, so after explaining the rules to Richard, I started in...

"You respond code 3 to a fifty year-old female found unresponsive. You arrive on-scene and the fire department is doing CPR. Take it from there. Anything you ask will be answered."

"Ok, is it summer or winter? Is there any family I can ask what happened?"

"It is summer and the house is air conditioned. The family members say they came home and found her on her bed with an empty bottle of pills. They were unable to wake her and called 911."

"Ok, what is the medication that was in the empty bottle?"

"Verapamil."

"Ok, I stop CPR, while I have my partner put the patient on the monitor and check for a pulse."

"You have a pulse of 42 bpm."

"Good, is she breathing?" "Yes, 4 to 5 respirations a minute. She is sinus bradycardia on the monitor, corresponding with pulses at 42 bpm."

"Good, I have the fire department hold on chest compressions and have them continue assisting respirations. What is her blood pressure?"

"78/50."

"Ok, I start an IV and administer .5 mg of atropine and 10mg of Calcium Chloride."

"The patient's heart rate is now 80 bpm and her blood pressure is 122/82."

"Ok, is she still unconscious? And what are her respirations?"

"She is still unconscious, and her respirations are 4-5 per minute."

"Alright, I intubate with a 7.0 ET tube and continue assisting respirations. I head to the nearest hospital code 3."

"Alright, when you get to the hospital and give report the doctor, he asks you if there were any other medications she might have taken."

"Oh shit, she had a narcotic overdose as well. I should have checked for other medications and checked her pupils, then administered Narcan"

Verapamil is a Calcium Channel Blocker used to control and slow down the heart rate of patients. Obviously if taken in excess, it causes an extremely slow heart rate. In any drug overdose, the paramedic needs to consider any other medications or substances that may have been consumed.

As the summer continued on, Little Brother and I got called to respond Code 3 to Brandel Manor Nursing and Convalescent Care, which was across the street from Emanuel Medical

Center. Emanuel's ER was on diversion due to an overload of patients so they were only open to Code traffic. When we arrived at Brandel Manor, we were directed to room 102 where we found an 88 year-old female who was unconscious and unresponsive. The staff told us that the patient was a no code, which meant no CPR or shocking could be done. The nursing staff also added that the patient had a medical history of stroke and is normally nonverbal. However, they stated that she was usually sitting up and looking around. The staff gave us the transfer paperwork which I scanned to check for any other medical problems the patient might have, along with any medications she was on or known allergies. Brian gave me the blood pressure, 78/52 and a pulse of 130 bpm with respirations of 36. He then put her on the EKG monitor, which showed sinus tachycardia. After listening to her lungs, which I heard upper rhonchi and diffuse sounds over the left lower lobe. Combining this with the fact that the patient was hot to touch and when squeezing the skin on her wrist it stays in place, I determined that she probably had pneumonia. Obviously, this was not something that happened overnight, but with the amount of patients the staff monitors, this was not uncommon. Brian and I loaded up the unconscious patient, whom I believe had a deadly pneumonia, and headed for the ambulance. Brian set up a bag of IV solution while I strapped a tourniquet around the patients arm and looked for an IV site. I missed my first attempt with an 18ga in her left wrist and Brian asked if I wanted to try the smaller 20ga. In the field, we try to start an 18ga on medical patients since it is the smallest needle that blood can pass through and attempting to administer medications through something smaller can be tedious.

I told Brian that I am going to take a shot at the patients left ac first and, luckily, I caught a flash in the angio catheter chamber on my second attempt. Attaching the IV tubing and taping it in place, I started a 250cc fluid bolus to see if I could increase the patient's blood pressure and decrease her pulse rate. As Brian jumped up front to drive, he reminded me that Emanuel was on diversion. I told him to turn on the med-net radio and hit the lights; we would transport code 3. I called the hospital with my code 3 report and advised them we were less than one minute out, just across the street at Brandel Manor. When we brought the patient in, I could see we were not going to receive a warm welcome. The charge nurse asked me, "Don't you know we are diversion?" I replied, "Yes, but this is a code 3 patient." The ER physician blurted out, "This is ridiculous! That's not a code 3 patient; you are incompetent." I pushed the gurney aside. Shaking my head with my eyes narrowed, I approached the physician and squared off with him. "Are you saying that I am incompetent, or are you saying that all paramedics are incompetent?" "I am saying you, and all of them are incompetent", he replied. I looked him in the eye as the whole emergency room became silent. I told him, "That's funny, doctor, because I, and the rest of the paramedics, think the same of you." We brought the patient into room 1 where the seriously sick and injured are placed and gave report to the nurse who was accepting the patient. I explained that while the patient was a no code, this was a new onset of unresponsiveness. The patient's pulse rate was fast and her blood pressure was low. That, along with the other symptoms led us to assume that she has an unmanaged pneumonia. I never heard any complaints about my confrontation with the physician, and we actually became good friends after that. I knew he was just blowing off steam and that they were overloaded in the ER. But hey, don't shoot the messenger.

Two weeks earlier, we had responded Code 3 to one of the local convalescent homes. Upon arrival, the staff told me that the patient, a lady in her seventies was unresponsive and they believed she had a stroke. I asked how long the patient had been like that. They told me she passed out while sitting at the lunch table. I ask "Ok, does she have any other medical conditions, such as diabetes?" The nurse replied "Yes, she is diabetic." Jeremiah, my partner on this day, placed the patient on oxygen and set up the glucometer. When I got the glucose reading, I saw that it was 24 mkg/kg, which is extremely low (a normal reading is between 70 to 100)—problem solved. We decided to load the patient into the ambulance and work her in the unit, as opposed to doing that in the patient's room. At this point she had been hypoglycemic for hours. The patient passed out around noon and it was now 3 p.m. We loaded her on the gurney and as we passed the nurses station we were asked by a staff member if the patient was going to be alright. Jeremiah put his head down next to the patients and in a shrill voice said "no I am not alright, my glucose is dangerously low". The staff nurses eyes widened as I added, "don't worry the state department will be investigating" Jerimiah and I were almost in tears, trying to keep from laughing. Once we passed the nurses station, I stopped the gurney and walked back and told the nursing assistant we were just teasing, everything was fine. In the ambulance, an 18ga angio catheter in the patient's left hand was hooked up to a bag of Normal Saline, followed by 25 grams of Dextrose 50% IV. The would-be stroke patient (according to the nursing home) is now fully awake and talking.

Chapter 12

June 12, 1993

I was working in Turlock with Chuck McCoy, who went through the second paramedic class in 1974. The owner of Turlock Ambulance, Roy Hirschkorn, had attended the first program. Chuck was not only an excellent paramedic, but he had an ability to consume knowledge, and then years later, bring it forward verbatim and with complete understanding. He was the manager of Turlock Ambulance and our softball team as well. Chuck and I were working a shift and had just dropped a patient off at Emanuel. We were busy changing the sheets on the gurney when Anne, one of the new Respiratory Therapists at the hospital, asked me how I liked being a paramedic. I answered that it was a challenge at times, but I enjoyed it when a life hung in the balance. She told me that she had thought about being a paramedic, so I told her that she should come and check it out with Chuck and myself. "Really, I can come along with you guys", She asked, thinking I was joking. "Here, this is the number for our dispatch. Call and tell them you have our approval, and set up a time that is convenient for you." Anne Marie Fontana was her full name and she showed up to ride with us for an evening shift the following week. As usual, when a rider comes along, we were blessed with a quiet evening. When the morning came, Anne and I met for breakfast. This was the beginning of a new Wednesday morning regime. The next week at work, Chuck and I ran a cardiac arrest and brought it into Emanuel ER where Anne was the attending Repertory Therapist. She was extremely competent and to really enjoyed her work. Of course she ribbed us about not getting a good call when she was riding with us.

I took on another student named Mike Rehan. He was a big friendly guy who was eager to learn and even more eager to please us. His first call was in Keys, just South of Turlock. The old part of Keyes is a small town with dirt walkways in front of the houses instead of sidewalks. It was a well-known area for welfare recipients and drug trafficking.

We loaded the gurney with our equipment, and made our way into the small, disarrayed house, where we were greeted by family members who were screaming that the patient, a 30 year-old female, was not breathing. Walking up to the patient in the cigarette smoke filled room, I deferred to Mike to take over. Mike asked what happened and was told that the patient had stopped breathing, so they started CPR. Reaching for a pulse and finding one, but noticing the patient was not breathing, Mike grabbed for the Ambu-bag and was about to start ventilating the patient. I, having noticed that the patient was nice and pink, stopped him. He gave me a strange look, so I told him to try talking to her first. Mike asked the patient what her name was with no reply and turned to me again. This time I told him to try rubbing her sternum. When he did, the patient sat up, coughing and swinging at him. As it turned out, the patient had been in a verbal disagreement when she started coughing violently and supposedly stopped breathing.

Mike asked me, after the patient refused transport and signed the AMA (against medical advice) paperwork, how I knew. I replied that the patient had no apparent past medical problems to attribute for not breathing, and her color was good. I told Mike that you cannot always take the patient's reported symptoms at face value. More often than not, alcohol or drugs were involved.

Anne and I became increasingly closer. She was going through a divorce, and I was on the mend from my last relationship. We decided to take a day trip to Santa Cruz and hung out on the boardwalk. Later, we rolled into Capitola for a swim at the beach. When we walked into the surf, we both fell in and started laughing like crazy. We ran back to our blanket and I held it up over both our heads. As I stopped laughing for a second, I asked her how long we were going to go on like this. We embraced each other closely, and a quick kiss was all it took for me to be forever in love.

Mike Rehan had the internship of a lifetime; every code 3 call possible came his way. One day, just after lunch, we were called for a vehicle vs. pedestrian. Mike was pumped up and ready to go when we got to the scene of the call. The patient was a male, about 25 years of age, and was struck at about thirty-five miles per hour, causing him to fly about twenty feet and land on the pavement. He was breathing with some difficulty and asking what happened? Mike did a quick head to toe exam after first getting a radial pulse that was thready and talking with the patient, which ascertained his airway was intact. The patient had an obvious left femur fracture and multiple abrasions and bruises. Mike lead the firemen in getting the patient immobilized on the backboard while cutting away clothing. The driver of the car that struck the patient was fine and refused treatment. Once inside the ambulance with the patient, Mike placed him on oxygen and had his EMT place the patient on the EKG monitor. I was third person, watching over Mike and taking notes on what to talk about later. I would not intervene unless it was life or death; this was the student's time to learn, and helping him work on the patient does not encourage learning. Mike's patient had a pulse rate of 136 and blood pressure of 98/60. The monitor was now hooked up and showing sinus tachycardia corresponding with pulses at 136 bpm. Mike's EMT, who happened to be Brian, set up two bags of Normal Saline upon Mike's request. I continued to watch, smile, and nod my head in approval, and try my best not to intimidate Mike. Mike settles in to start an IV, and I turn to Brian and said, "Let's go." Mike needed to do this en-route. Brian replied "Ok, code 2 or 3?" Mike spoke up, "Code 3; thanks." Mike got the IV with a 14ga in the patient's right arm and was getting prepared for the next IV when the patient stated he could not breathe. I listened to the patient's lung sounds and noticed that they were severely diminished on the right side. So without a word to Mike, I handed him the stethoscope and he listened. Mike asked me what I thought, and I returned his question, "What do you think?" "I think his right lung sounds are decreased" I replied, "I agree. Tell me the procedure." "Insert the catheter over the second to third rib, mid clavicular line." "Ok, go for it." Mike told the patient that he was going to feel a poke in his chest and inserted the 12 ga between his ribs as air came rushing out of the catheter. Mike was sweating big time and looked up at me; I had a big smile on my face, "Strong work, Mike."

After dropping the patient off at the trauma center, we had a talk about the call. Mike was excited and on top of the world. I explained to Mike that you can never second guess yourself; the patient was tachycardic, borderline hypotensive, and complaining about shortness of breath. While the fast heart rate could have been due to the fractured femur or internal bleeding, you have to address the fact that the patient is having difficulty breathing. Every call is not text book, where you are going to find crepitus, subcutaneous emphysema, and a late sign of tracheal shift. Worst-case scenario, you decompress a patient's chest that does not need it. If you hold off, a patient can die.

Anne and I were now inseparable. We went camping, lifted weights, trained karate. We we're always on the go, from surfing in Capitola at 41st street to concerts in Lake Tahoe. At Emanuel Hospital they called us Ken and Barbie since you would never see one without the other. I had met her Dad, Bob, and her step-mom, Gail, who treated me like family. We traveled up to Eureka to see her mother and mother's boyfriend, and while we were there we camped out in Trinidad. We bought a crab trap at an indoor flea market and set out for crabbing off the pier in Eureka. We caught dozens of Dungeness crabs, packed them on ice, returned to my father's house in Pleasant Hill, and had a crab fest.

One weekend we took off with Steve (Bucky) and his girlfriend, Jill, to Monterey. We found a hotel with a pool and hot tub, and rented a room. After a glass of wine and relaxing in the hot tub, we decided to take a spin down to Lover's Point Beach. We walked about the beach and then across the street to the Old Bath House restaurant and bar. The restaurant was so overfilled we could not get a table, so we found ourselves in the bar. We ordered Mud Slides, which is a concoction of Kahlua, Baileys, and vodka blended into a smoothie. Two Mud Slides later, we jumped into Jill's Chevrolet four-wheel drive truck. With Steve driving we headed back for the hotel, only we did not make it there. We were passing a park, where the police had a car pulled over at the curb. Bucky was looking at the police car and almost missed a stop sign, causing us to skid to a stop. The sirens and flashing lights now behind us, Steve was pulled over and arrested for a DUI. Steve made it back to the hotel in a taxi the following morning. Jill called her mother, who is an attorney, to take the case since you cannot work as a paramedic if you have a DUI. Steve managed to get the hearing postponed several times before appearing and being found guilty.

Chapter 13

Mike Rehan was still riding third person with me, and trying to finish up his internship. My partner was Troy Hirschkorn, who was just accepted into the Air Force Para Rescue training program. We were just delivering a patient to the ER in Turlock when we heard the familiar address of a patient go out over the radio. "Medic 202, respond code 3 to 1100 Alpha Road, apartment number 54 for an 83 year-old female with chest pain." This was a regular, or frequent flyer, who called every week complaining of either chest pain or abdominal pain in search of pain medication. You would not think an 83 year-old would fake symptoms until you met Harriet Lazotte. She would fake unconscious for the chance to get a ride to the hospital.

I once brought Harriat into the ER to a new agency nurse. Agency nurses are outsourced so the hospital does not have to hire new nurses or pay overtime, but of course the agency nurses are paid almost double and have no clue as to how things work when they first begin. I had never seen this nurse before. She looked at me, yawning, and asked, "Ok what have you got?" I had already told the patient that she should play dead when the nurse checks on her, for a little fun. I told the nurse that the patient had a run of ventricular tachycardia, so we administered 25 grams of Dextrose. I said the patient had a cardiac history, and we could not get a blood pressure. As I looked at Harriet and winked, I told the new nurse, "I think the patient just stopped breathing." The nurse looked at Harriet, who was perfectly still, holding her breath, and she then called another nurse and told her, "We have a code blue." She then glared at me and said, "The patient was in ventricular tachycardia and you gave her D-50?" "Yeah, I held up a box of D-50 and continued, it's the blue box, right? I think she needs another one." The nurse is now looking at the paramedic patch on my arm with a confused look on her face. About that time, the charge nurse, Carlyon Moeller, walks over and looks at me with a smile, and then at Harriet. She tells Harriet, "Open your eyes now, if you want me to treat you." Harriet opened her eyes and took a deep breath with a smile on her face. I looked at the agency nurse and said, "I'm sorry, just having a little fun. Welcome to Turlock."

Troy and I looked at each other, as the ambulance that was responding was about a mile further away than we were. Troy asked, "Do you want to take it? It's Harriet and Mike has not met her." "Ok," I said, "Just don't tell him we go out there every week. Let's see how he does." We radioed dispatch that we would handle it. When we arrived at the call, I told Troy to bring in the equipment with Mike. "I am going to catch up with the fire department and tell them not to let the student know we come out here all the time." Mike came in with Troy, walked up to the patient to take a pulse and asked what the problem was. Harriet replied "I am having chest pain." "What does it feel like?" Mike asked. "It feels like chest pain." "Ok, when did it start?" "Two years ago, can you give me something?" Mike is getting frustrated, since every question he asked leads nowhere, "Are those your medications", Mike asked as he pointed to the nightstand. The firemen handed Mike the medications, and Mike asked if another medication on the other night stand was hers. As he was reaching for it, Harriet screamed and deftly grabbed the medication before Mike could get to It. "That is mine! The doctor gave that to me and you can't have it." Mike asked "Ok, can you tell me what it is?" "It's mine, you can't have it, that medicine is for pain." Mike got a set of vitals which are: blood pressure 82/64, a pulse of 182 bpm, and respirations of 18. After placing the patient on oxygen at 6 liters by nasal cannula and attaching the patient to the EKG monitor, Mike had Troy set up an IV bag of Normal Saline and started an 18ga angio catheter in Harriet's upper left arm. The firemen and Troy loaded the patient onto the gurney and we all headed for the ambulance. Once in the ambulance, the fire department was ready to leave when I told them to hang around for a minute, because you are going to want to see this. Mike, who is inside the ambulance, asked me if the EKG rhythm was supraventricular tachycardia, or rapid atrial fibrillation. I asked him if it was regular or irregular. "Irregular", he stated, "It's atrial fibrillation, do you want me to give Verapamil?" "Well, since the patient is having chest pain, and their blood pressure is low, this would be considered unstable." "You want me synchronize cardiovert her." "Sounds good to me, but it is your choice." Mike put the gel on the paddles and set the EKG monitor to synchronized mode. He placed the paddles on Harriet's chest and told her she was going to feel a little shock. Mike set the power to 100 joules and shocked the patient. Harriet's heart rate dropped to 78 bpm and was now a normal sinus rhythm. Harriet started hyperventilating and suddenly let out a loud scream, "You, you, you tried to, to kill me!" Mike answered, "No, ma'am. I just saved you." When we got to the hospital, the nurses were all hugging Mike and laughing themselves silly. I showed the EKG to Dr. Craig, who looked at it and said, "Good job." Harriet did not call 911 for months after that.

Chapter 14

December 28, 1995

Anne and I were now living together. We had been bouncing back and forth between her home and mine, and when were off of work, we headed out for the coast or the mountains. Anne and I had rented a condominium at Mountain Retreat in Arnold for our Christmas, since we had to work the holidays. This would be our own celebration. We had done the same thing for the last two Christmases, and would have my kids, Sarah and K.C., and her parents up to celebrate and go skiing. I was on the end of 60-hour Shift, and Anne had gotten off earlier that night. We planned to leave in the morning for our seven-night stay.

The phone rang at 3 am; it was our dispatch wanting to know if they could give our crew's quarters phone number out to Mercy Ambulance in Coulterville (Mercy had beaten Riggs out of the county contract 5 years later). I worked occasionally for Mercy, so I figured they were hurting for a medic in the morning. When the phone rang and I answered it, it was one of the guys I worked with up there. He told me Anne had been in an accident, and her car ran off the road down a cliff. "I'm sorry, Bill, she did not make it." It was unbelievable; I hung up the phone and screamed, punching the wall. Troy came into my room, asking what was going on. I told him while I was packing up my gear to leave. Troy said he would call the supervisor; I really did not give a shit. I needed to call her parents, but I did not have their phone number, so I drove out to their house and rang the doorbell at 4:00 in the morning. The unbelieving look in her parent's eyes and the repetitive, "Tell me you are joking" still haunts me. Before I left Anne's parents' house, I called Little

Brother and, waking him up, I gave him the news. He said "I'll meet you out in front of my house in twenty minutes." I drove over to Brain's; he had duffel bag of clothes and his sleeping bag. I had a large bottle of Seagram's 7 that Anne's dad gave me, and we headed for her house. I drank and drank, wandering around the property. Anne's grandpa had forty acres of almonds, and there were five houses on the property. I did not eat or sleep for three days. Brian stayed by my side the whole time, answering phone calls and shielding me from all the well-wishers whom I could not bear to talk with or see. The funeral was set for five days later, as it was coming up on the weekend, I begged Anne's parents to keep the casket closed, since I could not bear to see her not alive, which they did. I went to the funeral home every day leading up to the funeral, and I sat in a side chapel that overlooked the casket. On the third day, Brian got a hold of Dr. Craig and had a prescription filled with sleeping pills. That night, after seeing her parents, I finally ate and slept. Brian took me shopping for a new suit, and I felt as all time was standing still. American Medical Response had just bought Turlock Ambulance about six months earlier. I was on vacation for one week, but they gave me an extra week off. My ambulance partners and coworkers showed up the day of the funeral and, per my request, all wore Turlock Ambulance uniforms and sat in separate area, forty strong. When the casket was walked down the aisle, all forty plus ambulance personnel were lined up outside, side by side and with a salute. It was beautiful; the chapel was overfilled with standing room only. Anne always had a smile on her face and loved everyone, and everyone was there to pay their respects. When I went back to work, I would hear people complaining about trivial things and I found it to be so superficial. Had these people no idea of what is important in life? I would cry when songs came on the radio that reminded me of us. About a week after returning to work, Brian and I got a call for a motor vehicle rollover on South Bound Hwy 99. It was two girls, the same ages as Anne. The driver was trapped in the car, and the passenger had two broken legs. Little Brother came over to me as I stood dumbfounded on the highway and told me the twenty-six year-old female driver was dead. I just needed to go confirm it. I looked at Brian with tears in my eyes, saying nothing. He said that he would get it done.

I tried hard to be a better paramedic by offering a hand to the drunks and drug abusers, instead of giving them verbal hell. I would check in on the patients I transported the next time I brought a patient in, and would ask the families if I could get them some coffee or water. I would ask every elderly woman her name and where she was born. Their eyes would light up. I would ask if they were married, and usually they would answer that their husband had passed, so I would ask them what their husband did for a living. I would say that while I understand it is not a consolation, no man wants to bury his wife. He would rather have it this way and, in the blink of an eye, I believe we will all be together again.

I found myself unable to move anything around the house; I had to have everything just the way Anne left it. Gail came over one day with a truck, and started loading up Anne's clothes to give away. I tried to stop her, and she firmly told me, "Billy, she is not coming back." Anne's birthday crept up on me and. I found myself booking the same room at Manuel Mill Lodge, a bed and breakfast in Arnold. It had six rooms and a large, open lodge that looked out over a large deck and 3-acre lake. After leaving there, I went to Slick Rock and camped in the same spot we had the year before; I was having a hard time letting my best friend go.

Chapter 15

Back at work, I was once more with Little Brother and he always had my back. He was surprised to see my new interest in treating patients so compassionately, but somehow I think he understood that I was fulfilling a promise to myself. We were working Medic 201 when we got called to the Foster Farms Chicken plant for a man with a hand injury. Brian was extremely quiet as we went en-route, and I being his best friend, knew why. Little Brother suffered an industrial accident after getting out of the Navy, while working for Lockheed and Murrieta Missiles in Sunnyvale. Brian, who was Ex-Navy, was fast-tracking a Fire Department job at the base while continuing his education. Brian was working with a fifty-thousand ton break press one day, when a part became lodged. He instinctively reached to free it, when the press came down on his right hand. Little Brother spent an entire six months as a patient at Ralph K. Davies in San Francisco where Dr. Harry Bunkie tried every possibility to save his right thumb and index finger. The reattachment did not work after months of micro surgeries and hyperbaric treatments. Dr. Bunkie next wanted to try a toe to thumb transplant, for which he was the leader and most successful in the field. The toe to thumb would allow Brian to have the ability to perform as a fireman. Another six months of surgeries, treatments, and living in the hospital were carried on. Ultimately, the toe to thumb transplant did not take. Brian got a pretty bad case of deja vu whenever we ran injuries involving the hands, and rightfully so. Brian was a young man when he had his future career as a fireman taken away, and I am sure that the disfigurement, as well as the handicap, at such a young age was devastating. Brian had to learn to become dominant with his left hand, which is no easy task.

When we arrived at the Foster Farms plant, the Turlock Police Department was on-scene and, recognizing Officer Steve Hamil, I told Brian to hold tight one minute. I waved Steve over, asking if he would be my partner for minute so I could keep Brian out of it. Steve, who knew us both well and having worked the ambulance himself years earlier, always enjoyed helping out and replied, "Not a problem; let's go." We took the gurney and equipment into the plant and were directed over to a conveyer belt with a man caught up to his right shoulder in the belt. The patients hand was lying on the ground, still attached, but three feet beneath him. Turlock City Fire Department was already there with firemen Kain Packwood and Kirk Summers. Kain assured me that the conveyer belt was locked out and safe for us to approach. I approached the patient and had a Spanish-speaking coworker translate for me that we were going to get him out of there. And that I would be getting him something for pain shortly. I deferred to Kain and Kirk; any teaching to be done this day was going to be by them, as they were the extrication specialists. It became obvious that the patient was not going to come out easily, and Kain was thinking maybe if we could reverse the belt manually, we could free the patient that way. I asked Steve to go fetch Brian; I was going to need him. When Brian got there, he was all business and set up an IV bag of Normal Saline. He grabbed a white hospital towel and the interpreter, while he slid in behind the patient under the conveyor belt. Brian used the towel as a tourniquet around the patient's upper shoulder to control bleeding. Kain and Kirk tried manually releasing the belt and it moved forward instead of backward, so we had to scratch that idea. Brian told the interpreter to tell the patient that he would be right beside him until he comes out. I started a 16ga angio catheter in the patients left arm and administered Morphine for pain. Kain was not a happy fireman, we had been there for going on an hour and he was now going to try and cut the conveyor belt system apart. It was heavy-duty, forged metal with roller tracks. I called for a helicopter, figuring if and when we got the patient out he should be flown to the hospital if there was any chance of reattachment.

The cutting was going slow, so I conferred with Little Brother as to what he thought about amputation to get the patient free. Brian felt that there were only a few inches of muscle that were holding the arm in place. I called the hospital and apprised them of the situation and the need for a surgeon to amputate. They initially seemed to think that I was overreacting. I thought to myself, *they should know better, I always try to down play situations not the other way around*. We are rolling into the second hour, and the police department now has two units on-scene; they want to know what I need. I explained the situation and told them that at this point, the safest bet was to amputate a small amount of remaining muscle to get the patient free. I advised them I was going to need a surgeon or a physician for this, and hearing this they prepared to go arrest the base station physician if need be, and bring him on site. There is a general feeling of helplessness as we wait for the fire department to get the massive conveyor belt disabled. The police department drives over to Emanuel Hospital, and states they need to get a physician or surgeon out there now or people are going to start getting arrested. The police department returned code 3 with Dr.Hoak who was a general surgeon, a respiratory therapist, and a surgical Tech. I greeted the doctor and staff and gave them the run-down on the situation, including vitals and drugs administered. The surgeon piggybacked in Propofol (a milky white substance for conscious sedation), and cut the arm below the shoulder, freeing the patient. Brian was holding pressure with the towel as we placed the patient onto the gurney. As he released pressure, several arteries started spurting blood. Brian tightened his grip as Dr.Hoak cauterized several arteries and sutured the ones that refused to clot. Meanwhile, the patient had gone limp from the trauma, medications, and hours of being trapped. I assisted ventilations and the patient was intubated as we headed out to the helicopter. All in all, we were on-scene for three hours. It should have been at least only half of that, but for some reason our need for a surgeon to amputate was not taken seriously.

People often think of us as heroes, and I am not so sure that is true, at least not in my case. I have a job to do and I simply try to do it the best I can. I don't think we know who a real hero is until that moment it happens. The hero ends up being a regular person just like all of us, who reacts without regard for himself or without fore or afterthought. A simple reflex to put themselves in harm's way for a chance to save another's life.

I remembered about a year or so after losing Anne, my best friend, Victor, asked me to come up to Reno and be in his wedding, I really did not feel up to it, but he told me I did not have a choice since I was the best man. Victor and I met at about four years of age on View drive where we both lived in San Leandro, Ca. Victor, aka JAWS (his call sign in the Air Force), was an F-15 fighter pilot during the late 80's and early 90's. Victor ended up as a Red Flag Instructor, which is the Air Force's version of the Navy's Top Gun. When I talked to Vic before the wedding, I told to him that he got out just in time, as the Gulf War started about six months after his seven-year term. He replied, "Billy, you don't understand. I want to be there." Wow, it was hard to comprehend those words. That is one definition of a hero to me. Another is a man or woman who toils their life at work to support the family, and gives up any dreams once had so that their family may have a better life. There are a lot of heroes out there, and they don't always wear a uniform.

The patient at Foster Farms ended up losing his arm, despite all our efforts. I believe the hero that day was Little Brother.

One of the nice things about American Medical Response was that they received a contract to handle Yosemite National Park, and it was scheduled out of the Turlock Operations. Most of the paramedics did not want the extra drive, so it went to employees with less seniority. One paramedic who was fairly new was Clayton Ogden. He and I switched one sixty-hour shift a month, so he could run more calls in Turlock and I could enjoy the majesty of Yosemite. Working in Yosemite was like being on vacation. The best part was when a transfer out of the Valley, a Mercy Ambulance, would handle it from either Coulterville or Mariposa. The American Medical Response unit was dedicated to stay in the park, so being the AMR\Yosemite unit meant that our patients were taken either to the clinic for evaluation and release or flown out by helicopter and occasionally transferred out by Mercy Ambulance. I, while working for Mercy Ambulance had, on more than one occasion, the displeasure of transporting from the clinic to Fresno, which is not a fun drive. It is a long and twisty transport. The life-threatening calls were helicoptered-out, which was always a spectacular scene to watch.

I worked with either Terry Hirschkorn or George Maroudas. George was one of my students and was always a pleasure to work with. We had a small, two bedroom quarters on the back side of the clinic, and we would barbeque with the clinic doctors and nurses. We never had to go more than a mile or two into the park hiking after a patient, since the park had paramedic rangers and, of course, a search-and-rescue team to get the patients to us. During the day, we were supposed to help out in the clinic, but we pretty much always found an excuse not to be there. Dr. Kidd was one of the full-time doctors at the clinic, and enjoyed climbing on his days off. He was a young physician who had traditional ways and an easy-going nature. A patient in his 30's came in one day with an obviously dislocated shoulder, and before getting all the way checked in, Dr. Kidd evaluated him and gave him a shot of Xylocaine in the shoulder. He had me pull traction the opposite way while he reduced it. The nurses were a little troubled that the patient did not have an x-ray first, but Doctor Kidd said to simply take the x-ray now to assure it was back in proper place.

George and I ran some pretty good calls, including a cardiac arrest and several other trauma patients we had to fly out. I was leaving work one day when a seventy year-old lady was doing a three hundred-foot base jump to celebrate her birthday, and the chute never deployed. There was not much we could do for her.

On duty in downtown beautiful Turlock once again with Little Brother, we got a call that I will never forget. People always want to know what the worst thing is that you have ever seen, Well, we've seen the human body crushed, burnt, decapitated, and every imaginable horror possible. It was just a matter of how much time you spent on the streets. We were called out to one year-old male with CPR in progress. These types of calls come in all the time, and usually they are for a simple febrile seizure. Infants who are two years of age or less do not have a fully-developed hypothalamus, which controls heat regulation, and the seizure is not so much caused by the fever, but how and quickly it spikes. The treatment is to simply undress the child and remove any blankets that the mother may be using to cover the shivering baby. Sometimes we will do some simple cooling measures with a damp cloth and give blow by oxygen. It is, of course, possible that there are other underlying problems, and the infant continues to seize, so we then administer valium. The other less common reason for a child not breathing and "CPR in progress" is Sudden Infant Death Syndrome.

On this particular call, it was none of the above. When arrived at a chiropractor's office, the fire department was calling my name loudly, which was not a good sign. I walked in with Brian and saw them doing CPR on an infant who appeared to blue and mottled with skin sloughing off. Brian attached the EKG monitor quickly and it was asystole, flat line. Everyone was in a panic and the tension was high. I had Little Brother bring the baby to the ambulance so we could transfer to the hospital. I told the firemen that the child was gone, but we were going to transport to the hospital for the benefit of the parents. With the infant on the stretcher in back of the ambulance, I asked Brian to hit the lights and go. I looked at the child with a feeling of helplessness. I kept checking to make sure there were no signs of life, but it appeared that the little one was beyond our help hours ago. I called the hospital and updated them I was inbound with a deceased infant. I radioed that there would be a large crowd behind us and asked them to have security and a Chaplin ready. Bringing the baby to the hospital didn't make us any friends with the ER, but had we stopped CPR in front of the nearly dozen people, it would only have been worse. In the best interest of the parents, I wanted to give them the opportunity to grieve in a controlled environment where they could receive compassion.

The mother of the infant usually took the toddler to daycare in the mornings, however because she was running late, the father took the baby this day. When the mother went to pick up the infant at daycare that late afternoon, she found the toddler was not there and called the father at work. The father at first thought his wife was fooling with him. Then it hit him. He raced to his black Chevrolet Tahoe in the parking lot and found the lifeless toddler in the child seat still buckled in. It was a summer day in the hundreds on that fateful day and the infant was in the vehicle for eight hours. The worst thing I have ever seen was the mother's look on her face when Brian and I were taking her infant to the ambulance.

The media was outraged as the news hit the papers; the county child protective services filed criminal charges. My partner and I, along with the firemen, saw and felt what had happened; it was the worst kind of mistake that could be made. The father and mother were a solid Christian family. The father, who had work on his mind, didn't usually take the toddler to daycare and simply forgot. How much more punishment than losing your child and knowing it was your fault can befall a man? The charges were finally dropped. American Medical Response sent a supervisor out to the hospital to check on Brian and I, and offered us critical stress debriefing, which was extremely thoughtful and kind, but sometimes it is just better to get back in the saddle and talk it out amongst ourselves.

Chapter 16

On a rainy evening in Turlock I was working the 203 car, our first twelve-hour ambulance. The other two ambulances, 201 and 202, were still on the 24-hour system. They had a 60-hour work week when, for the same pay, we only worked 42 hours each week. Seniority does have its benefits. We would take code 3 calls that were sent to other ambulances and we were a back-up when another ambulance was already dispatched. We were posted downtown so we spent a lot of time at Lyon's restaurant where we were served complimentary drinks, soups, and salads, and occasionally would help bus tables We would also kept an eye on any riff raff that found its way into the lounge.

My partner on this shift was Terry; he would tell you that he has been working on the ambulance for 46 years although he is only 45 years old. He gladly counts the time his mom was running calls for Turlock Ambulance Service while pregnant with him. His dad owned Turlock Ambulance Service at the time. He could be a strong EMT when he wanted to, but for the most part you had to keep Terry on a short leash or your job would be in jeopardy. We would catch a cardiac arrest call and when we were walking down the hallway with the gurney, Terry would suddenly start running. I asked Terry what he was doing and he would say, "I see levidity, quick!" He screams "Let's get there before the fire department starts CPR." We arrived the same time as the firemen and when cutting the patients shirt off, Terry is right in there rolling the patient on his, chanting "Its levidity, its levidity." I responded, "Sorry Terry, the patient has agonal respirations; we are going to work it."

On that particular rainy evening in Turlock, we were called to respond code 3 for a motor vehicle accident on Hwy 99 southbound. It was north of Shanks road and was three to four cars with possible pin-ins. When we arrived and I stepped out of the door of the ambulance, the first thing I saw was a friend of mine, Gilbert, who just happened to be driving home when a car went flying through the air past him. There were four cars with two pin-ins and another vehicle on fire. Terry and I did a quick head count. We already had one ambulance on the way and we called for two helicopters as well. Three of the seven patients were in critical condition. The first unit showed up just minutes after we did and a young paramedic wearing a blue helmet walked over to me. He told me we should set up a triage area and incident command. Since it was dark and raining, the Hwy shut down, and patients were trapped in the wreckage. I told him to take the two walking wounded to Emanuel and maybe we will set up a triage area and incident command next time. Right now I want to get these patients out of here and on their way to hospitals. The next ground ambulance was carrying my old friend and first partner, Bob Easter. He came over to me and asked what I had for him. I told him I wanted him to be in charge of extricating pin-ins and preparing them to be flown out. The on-duty field chief showed up and jumped in the front seat of the rig offering me a hand. I told him that the first helicopter just landed and took a small infant who had been pulled from the burning vehicle. I told him we still had two patients who were pinned in and Bob, his partner, and a paramedic intern were working on those. We had to call one more helicopter, as well as one more ground unit. Back in the rig with Mike Aldred, the crew chief, I was deciding, along with Stanislaus Control, where to place the four patients left. The second Medi-Flight helicopter had landed and they were assigned a sixty-year-old male who had just been extricated from being trapped. Bob and his team had the patient fully immobilized, a full set of vital signs taken, and one large bore IV started. The patient appeared to have a fractured femur and his chest was opened where recently sutured from a recent bypass. The patient had stable vitals, and he was alert and talking. The third helicopter gave us an ETA of ten minutes when Bob knocked on my window to tell me that the second helicopter crew wanted to set the fractured leg and RSI (rapid sequence intubate) the patient. I told Bob that the patient needed to get out of here now. He replied that he told this to the helicopter crew, but they thought they could do whatever they wanted. At this point we had sent two more stable c-spine patients out by ground, and were down to our last two patients. I approached the flight crew and told them I wanted this patient transported now because I have another helicopter getting ready to land. The nurse told me that she did not feel comfortable transporting the patient the way he was. I looked at Bob and asked him if he would have a problem transporting this patient by ground to the trauma center, and he said "No problem, say the word." The helicopter crew discussed it and took the patient as directed, although they were not happy. The third helicopter arrived and patiently circled waiting for the second helicopter to lift off. They then landed and happily transported the last patient, an approximately 30 year-old patient who was trapped. She was in and out of consciousness and had massive facial trauma with bleeding. The total time on-scene took fifty-four minutes, involved three critical patients, two pin-ins, and a total of seven patients.

About a month later, a complaint came in. It was from the helicopter nurse who was pushing for an investigation by the EMS agency. American Medical Response gave me a copy of her

PCR (patient care report), along with a letter she sent to the agency expressing her concerns.

I felt that if she had concerns, she could have simply called or met with me. We disagreed on a treatment plan, so I figured we could just agree to disagree, but she bypassed me and the company she worked for by sending a letter to the EMS agency on her own accord. In her pre-hospital report, the nurse mentioned my name in the treatment portion of the document. This is not only improper, but obviously not the place to document something other than treatment. She stated in her report to the EMS agency that she did not feel I fully understood the seriousness of the patient's condition. She also spoke of how the patient had to be rapid sequence intubated upon her arrival to the hospital and that the patient had a pneumothorax that required a chest tube. On the scene of the call she never mentioned that she was concerned the patient might have a pneumothorax. If that was the case, placing the patient on oxygen would have been the first step, followed by decompressing the chest--not RSI. The fact that the patient was intubated and his chest was decompressed at the ER is irrelevant to the fact that the patient was speaking in full sentences and not complaining of shortness of breath while we were on-scene. After arrival to the ER, if the physician decided to RSI the patient and decompress his chest, it would be totally appropriate in order to prepare the patient for surgery. If she would have expressed these concerns on-scene, I would have had no problem with the flight crew decompressing the patient's chest if needed. In fact, if she wanted to splint the fractured leg and RSI the patient, and he was the only patient on scene, I would have let her even though I did not agree. However, that was not the case. In a triage situation, you have to do the most good for all the patients involved. I was now required to write an incident report, and while I'm not usually one to point fingers, I never would have pushed the paperwork that could jeopardize a nurse's or paramedic's career.

When I realized that this was the path the nurse was attempting to set up, I called Ron Duran (Little Duck), who is one of the head EMS agency's personnel in Merced County. When I told him about the situation I was in, he asked exactly where the call was, and realized it was in Merced County. Ron said that this was his jurisdiction, not Mountain Valley EMS agencies. He said that he and Merced County would do the investigating. In the end, Merced County put a stop to the Mountain Valley Agency's investigation and did their own. I, of course, got my hand slapped for being rude to the nurse, who said I yelled at her. Well I guess I might have it was dark and raining and she had a flight helmet on. The Merced County investigation also felt that I should have considered a second landing zone. In an ideal world that would have been great, but our resources were very limited.

This reminded me of a call where a young female student at Cal State was thought to have had a seizure in class, during a final. We were told she had no medical history that they were aware of, and nobody had witnessed any seizure activity. They simply noticed her with her head down on the desk during the exam. After we examined her, we saw that she had not bitten her tongue or gone incontinent--both signs with a seizure. When we approached her, she had her head slumped on her desk and was refusing to speak. This was a situation where we had to place her on oxygen, take vitals, attach the EKG monitor, and check her glucose (which was normal). I was under the impression she was acting, and when we wheeled her into the hallway, I told her firmly that she needed to talk to us, but got no reply. I told her that her heart rate was fast, so if she was taking methamphetamines I needed to know. She sat up straight and said "Who the hell do you think you are? I don't take drugs, you are a son of a bitch!" Mission accomplished. Since the patient was not happy with me, I let my partner take the call. When we got to the hospital, the patient asked a nurse for my name and a phone number where she could file a complaint. About a week later, I heard that she had posted my name and some crazy ranting's on Craig's List and when I asked around, I learned that she had a history of giving false reports. A friend of mine found her on Facebook where she listed herself as a flight nurse, which she was not, since she was just starting her pre-nursing classes. She started harassing my supervisors over the phone and it appeared that I may need a restraining order on her; she also had multiple complaints and false complaints against the university police and Turlock PD. She was finally expelled from the University after being caught giving multiple false statements to a police officers.

Chapter 17

Into the Present 2010-2012

Still working in Turlock for American Medical Response, all shifts were now 12 hours long and a 42 hour work week. 3 days one week followed by 4 days the next. We had posting areas throughout the County were we sit in the ambulance and wait for calls. My partner for now was Matt Turpin, who did not talk much. Usually after a couple hours, I will open the conversation with "Are you hungry?" "Yep", he would reply. Matt liked McDonalds, Togo's, or Subway while I was still a taco truck coinsure, so we took turns. After eating one night, we got a transfer from Emanuel to a private residence. As we rolled over to the hospital, the system depleted and there was no ambulance available for Turlock. We arrived at the hospital and I asked Matt not to go on-scene until another unit got close enough to Turlock to cover. Dispatch called us and asked if they could show on-scene, I replied "Standby one." I walked into the ER, spoke with the charge nurse, Chrissie, and explained we had no units in town. I asked if the transfer could hold and she said "Of course, Bill. How about 20-30 minutes?" I answered, "Great, I appreciate it. I owe you one." Back out in the ambulance, I radioed dispatch and told them I had spoken to the ER, and they would hold on the transfer, a code 2, returning a patient to their residence. Dispatch advised me that the hospital would have to confirm that with them. Matt and I shook our heads because the cover unit was almost into Turlock when they got dispatched to a difficulty breathing call. They were closer than we were, but we still didn't have coverage for Turlock. The dispatch was now sending another unit to cover Turlock, but it was still in downtown Modesto, twenty minutes away. We next heard the unit that was coming to cover from Modesto got dispatched for a hanging two blocks away from us. Matt grabbed the radio and told them we were responding. When we arrived on-scene of the residence, the patient was in the garage with the door open. Two female police officers already had her on the ground and were performing CPR. I didn't have to tell Matt what to do, since we had been working together for over a year and had done this over and over. Matt placed the 40 year-old female on the EKG monitor and set me up a bag of Normal Saline as I intubated. She was in astoyle on the monitor, but we were going to continue with our efforts. With cardiac arrest patients, I like to start a 14ga angio cath in the external jugular vein. It is more central to the heart and will get the medications there faster. You can also run your IV at an incredible flow rate if needed. This is a skill that needs to be practiced regularly so you can do it without fail, even when the shit hits the fan. Also, I am already at the patient's head, making it easier than moving around to the patient's arms. The IV goes in easily, since the external jugular vein is large. We taped it in place and administered 1mg of Epinephrine and 1mg of Atropine while CPR was being continued. The EKG was still astoyle and while I knew the efforts were fruitless, we c-spined and back boarded the patient. We headed to the hospital with the help of the female police officers and the firemen who were doing compressions and ventilating, while I continued to push drugs and called the ER. The code was worked for about five minutes with no change in patient condition, and after arrival to the ER it was called.

We redeemed ourselves during the next shift when we were called out for CPR in progress at the Crane Park tennis courts. After loading up our equipment and rolling the gurney across the lawn to the tennis courts, we found the fire department doing CPR on a sixty year-old, fit male. The firemen told us that they had shocked him once and were continuing with CPR. After hooking up our monitor, the patient was in ventricular fibrillation. We shocked at 200 joules and continued CPR for a minute before rechecking the rhythm, which was SVT at 180 bpm. Matt felt a strong radial pulse as the firemen were checking for a blood pressure and assisting respirations since the patient was not breathing. I intubated the patient and Matt set up a line of Normal Saline, the fireman gave us a blood pressure of 190/90. I started the IV in the arm this time because the patient had ropes for veins. Mat was pointing at the monitor telling me "The patient is in SVT at 180; what do you want to do?" I replied that we were not going to mess with it and asked him to hand me two preloads of Lidocaine. I administered 150mg IV and we started to package the patient. I asked Matt to go to the unit and set me up a second IV and a Lidocaine drip. We loaded the patient into the ambulance and I then piggy backed the lidocaine drip into the first IV, and set it at 2mg a minute. We took off, code 3, for Emanuel Hospital and I had Matt call it in while I started a second IV. The patient's heart rate was coming down to 100 bpm and his blood pressure was now 140/80. In the hospital, the patient was now breathing on his own, following commands, and trying to talk. The son who was playing tennis with his father told us when we arrived that his dad walked over to grab a ball by the fence and collapsed. There was a nurse nearby, and she and the son performed CPR until the fire department arrived.

When Mat had his bachelor party, he just wanted to go to an air-show. A close knit group of about six EMS personnel met at Chad's house before going to the Beale Air Force air show. When we had all arrived at Chad's house, Chad came out with a t-shirt; he told Matt before we left he would have to change shirts. Chad gave Matt the t-shirt he had made two sizes too small. The shirt was a girly blue color with "I Love (the love was a big sparkly heart) Air shows" on the front, and on the back it said in bigger letters, "A Whole Lot." It looked hilarious when Matt put it on, it fit ridiculously tight, and the heart shimmered in the sun light. When we arrived at the air show, we promptly downed some cold beers from our cooler, since we did not know if alcohol was allowed or not. Matt actually had several people inquire as to where he got his shirt; they wanted one, too. The air-show was awesome, and afterward we took off for old town Sacramento. We ate dinner at Fanny Anne's Salon, followed by club hopping, and we ended up at a bar called "The Dive". The bar was packed shoulder to shoulder, and it was easy to get separated from the group. Michael Conover is 6'4" and wearing a large, black Stetson 24x cowboy hat. Eric Walthrop, a well sized young body builder, was wearing wranglers with Justin Roper boots, a white t-shirt, and a ball cap. Thirty minutes or so into our adventure at the Dive, and the bouncers told Eric he had to either take off his ball cap or leave. Eric was not about to take off his hat, so I located Conover by the top of his Stetson, bellied up to the bar and drinking Crown Royale. I told him we needed to leave or Eric would be thrown out because the bouncers wanted him to take off his hat. Conover, who is surrounded by girls looking like they wanted his autograph, told me, "Screw him, I'm staying," "No, Mike", I replied, "We came together and we stay together." He laughed as he downed his drink; we rounded up the guys and headed out for more clubs. Eric was huffy, saying he took his hat off for no one.

Chad had nicknamed Eric, Back Yard Billy as several months earlier he and Eric both had their vehicles windows busted out and their stereos stolen at the ambulance station one night.

While Chad had his Lexus window replaced and re-tinted the next day, Eric's window on his Dodge truck stayed broken for months, he said, "Hell, maybe I will fix it if it starts raining. Maybe."

We finally found a club that sounded inviting with its loud country music. We were all trying to get Matt drunk and kept his glass full at all times. Matt was not a drinker and on occasion he would drink Mikes Lemonade, which we all made fun of him for. After a couple of hours and a lot of alcohol, the band changed to some demonic, screaming music, and people started moshing on the dance floor. I hold my liquor well, and I was keeping an eye out for the group when I noticed that Conover was missing. I made my way through the crowd to find him wasted and moshing in the outer circle of the dance floor. He was shoving a large punk-rocker whose face was covered in piercings every time the punker turned away from him. I watched a few more shoves before corralling him up and we all got out of there.

Matt, or Turp as we call him, was as serious about his job as he was silent. He always went through every cabinet and every bag of equipment, and checked the dates on all the drugs every shift. Turp checked and calibrated the glucometer and checked all the monitor batteries at the beginning of each shift, as well. He would then turn on all the lights and walk around the unit checking the tires, and finished with a quick chirp of the siren.

On-duty and working the 206 unit in Turlock, Turp and I received called to a code 3 in Denair for a psychological disorder. We were given stand-back orders until cleared by the sheriff's office that was also en-route. Matt pulled up and parked a block away from the call, alongside the Denair

Volunteer Fire Department engine, and got out to talk with the firemen. As he was getting out, I saw a man walking strangely towards us and I told Turp, "That is our guy." He replied "No, this is not even the right street." Matt walked over to the firemen, and I got out of my side of the ambulance into the night, watching the stranger move toward me. As the man got closer, I noticed he was talking to himself, which is something I do a lot, except his arms were moving, making gestures, and then he would laugh. He was kind of meandering this way and that, so I was more than sure that this had to be our patient. As he got up to me, I said hello and he stopped. I told him we were dispatched out here for a person not feeling well, and asked if it was him. "Yes", he replied, and I motioned for him to follow me. I told him to jump into the back of the ambulance for a minute so I could get his blood pressure and check him out. I wanted him to go ahead of me for safety reasons, but he started to turn away, so I jumped in ahead of him and coaxed him along to follow me, asking his name and what I could do to help tonight. As he slid in, Matt came over to see what was going on and opened the second ambulance door. The man screamed and dashed out of the ambulance, "I think that's the patient, Turp." Before I could say another word, Matt took off after the guy, running like an Olympic gold medalist. I raced over and jumped into the ambulance, which was facing the wrong way, and turned it around in pursuit of my partner and patient. They were zigzagging from one side of the dark street to the other with Turp gaining ground quickly. As I finally caught up, the crazy guy had fallen to the ground. When I got out of the unit, Matt had his foot on the mad man's back yelling at him to stay down. As I approached the two, Matt took his foot off of the guy's back and said "I got him." "Good work, Turp. Just one thing, can you put your foot back on him?" Turp looked at me and said, "Sure." I clicked a picture with my phone camera. The guy was on meth and tried to kill his wife, the sheriff told us after he handcuffed the patient and placed him in the back of his patrol car. No problem Sheriff, my partner Turp here, had it all under control.

Of course, that was not the first time Officer Turp had been in pursuit. Early one morning, about 3 a.m. we were parked at a Valero gas station when a meth head started harassing customers and kicking their cars. Matt jumped out of the ambulance and yelled at the guy, "Hey, stop that; get out of here." The junkie started coming towards Turp, so I jumped out with my portable radio and called dispatch for police backup. He started to take a swing at Matt, but before he could make contact, Mat stepped forward and grabbed his arm. The would-be assaulter took off running down Golden State Boulevard with Turp on his heels. Again, I jumped into the unit and followed them across the street to the Woods Furniture store parking lot. Before the police arrived, two other Turlock ambulances slid into the parking lot code 3. Dave Murphy, who we all called Big Daddy, is 6'6" and a solid 350 lbs. The other ambulance had Robert Parker, who was 5'5" and 160lbs. Parker was an ex-military MP, built like a compact Sherman tank, and had a fireplug temper--always ready for a challenge. Big Daddy and Parker stepped out of their ambulances and surrounded Mr. Wannabe-tough guy, until the police arrived and arrested him.

Turp had a soft spot for young, tragic deaths, two of which I recalled that were motor vehicle accidents. The first was an automobile vs. train where a young girl of 18 years ran head-on into the side of the train. When we got to her, she was pinned into the car, not breathing, and had no pulse. I walked over to confirm her as DOA, and Turp asked me if we could do anything for her. I told him if she was not pinned in, then we could work her, but by the time Fire gets her out, it just was not going to happen. The second call was on Hwy 99, northbound, at Fulkerth road. It involved two vehicles and once again our patient was a young female, pinned inside her car without a pulse. Matt placed her on an EKG to confirm death, and I could sense how he did not like being unable to help her. It can be tough when you want to help but there is nothing to be done.

Mat moved to the day shift after getting married. My new partner was Chad. We worked on the 206 unit that was from 6 p.m. to 6 a.m. Chad was a new paramedic when we first start working together. He was brilliantly smart and had a bachelor's degree in teaching. He latter started flying for Reach Air Services, as well as prepared to enroll in the physician's assistant program.

Chad had an extremely dry sense of humor and quick wit, so most people don't pick up on the fact he is teasing with them. Trying to get the better of him with insults just does not work because he was always one step ahead. We enjoyed working together as he drilled me on all the latest protocols and laughed when I told him I run my calls without thinking about the protocols. I said if I have any doubts for the charting, then maybe I would check the protocols. Chad's pre-hospital reports were thorough and his penmanship was perfect, with times written on every line. He laughed at me because he said I was the only paramedic he knew who could chart a cardiac arrest call on less than half of report page. My times were always the same. I charted at the top when we'd made patient contact, drew a line to departure and another line to when we arrived at the hospital. Even funnier was that I cannot always read my own hand writing. Chad asked what I would say if the case ended up in court and I told him the less I wrote the less they could read, so much the better. I would decipher it as needed when the time comes. It's better to scribble like a physician and explain it properly when asked than have someone review your chart and question each minute you have listed on the report. Chad liked to test me on everything in the book; which was great for me. "What are the only two pediatric drugs with a dose of .03 mgs", he would ask me. I'd say, "I did not know we served Happy Meals on the ambulance; how about Atropine and Glucagon?" Chad replied, "There may be hope for you yet." There probably wasn't, since I was stuck in my ways. With Chad being the new paramedic, instead of rotating calls I took all the bullshit and let him have the occasional hot calls. He did know that if he hesitated on treatment I would jump in, so he was always giving me a look for approval. On one sweleringly hot night, we go called for a sick male at one of the local motels. When we arrived at the patient's room, the fire department was just pulling in. We walked into the room and found an oriental man who did not speak English in the extremely warm motel room. The patient was on the far side of the room, sitting on the bed. The firemen had crowded in to get vital signs as the patient was pointing to his chest saying something that sounded like "It's hot, it's hot." "Yeah, no shit; we are all sweating our asses off, pal", I murmured under my breath. The fire department said they were not able to get a good blood pressure because the patient was moving around too much. When we got him onto the gurney and placed the EKG monitor and the automatic blood pressure cuff on, we saw that he was in SVT at rate of 200 bpm. The blood pressure came in at 80/56, so Chad placed the defibrillator pads on (we no longer used paddles, but instead pads that would show the rhythm, and you would shock the patient like an AED). As we wheeled him outside into the fresh air, I asked Chad what his plan was. He stated, "Put him in the ambulance and get an IV going for starters." I replied, "You do realize he is unstable?" Chad stated "You want to cardiovert him now?" I replied, "Well, I want you to push the button or I will." Chad shocked the patient at 100 joules into a nice sinus rhythm. We now realized the patient was saying heart, heart vs. hot, hot. Once in the back of the ambulance, I set up a bag of Normal Saline and tore tape for Chad as he started the IV. The patient's blood pressure was now normal at 128/82. When we arrived at the hospital and were transferring the patient over to the hospital bed, one of the ER techs, that was helping us to transfer the patient, was chatting away, asking the patient questions, and not paying attention. The patient yelled, "I am Chinese, no speak English. Shut up." Chad and I looked at each other, suppressing our laughter until we got outside. Chad and I had a side-splitting laugh in the ambulance bay as we restocked and readied our ambulance. Chad asked me if I thought it might have been better to have an IV on the patient before cardioverting him. I replied "If the cardioversion did not work, he would either stay in the same rhythm, or in the worst case scenario, he would go into ventricular fibrillation. At that point we shock him again and if he did not convert, we start CPR. There is really no medication to push prior to shocking the patient, since he is unstable unless you want to risk starting an IV and sedating the patient first.

Chad and I picked up an overtime day shift one sweltering summer day, and were dispatched to the Home Depot parking lot for an unconscious patient. When we pulled into the parking lot, a Home Depot employee wearing an orange vest waved us over to a vehicle. The employee had the car door open and an elderly lady was slumped over. He told us that he found her slumped over in the front seat of the Honda Accord and he opened the door to check on her. The patient was truly unconscious, as reported. Chad knew this would be his call, since this looked like a real medical aid. He ascertained that the patient had a pulse by checking her radial artery at the wrist and assessed her breathing. We loaded the patient onto the gurney and lifted her into the back of our unit where it was comfortable and cool with the air conditioning running. Chad placed the patient on oxygen and grabbed the EKG monitor leads to apply, and then looked up at me as I poured a liter of bottled sterile water over the patients head and chest. His said, "Holy shit, I was going to place ice packs under her arm pits; can you do that?" The elderly lady opened her eyes and took a deep breath as I replied, "I Just did." Grabbing for a second liter of bottled sterile water, I continued pouring it over the rest of her body. Chad finished putting on the EKG monitor and got the patient's blood pressure as I spiked him an IV line and tore tape for him. The patient's blood pressure was 82/60 and her heart rate was 150 bpm, so after Chad established the IV, he started a fluid bolus and I drove to the hospital. After Chad had given the patient report to the ER and we were outside drying of the gurney, he asked me again, "Are you sure we can do that?" I replied, "I am not sure, but that's how I have been doing it for almost thirty years." Chad stated "I thought we needed to bring her temperature down slowly." "Well, if they are hypothermic we bring it up slowly, but in this case our patient is hyper-thermic and long past heat exhaustion, and she is now in heat stroke, which can be lethal. I once had a guy so far gone in his oven of a house, that we literally drug him out to the front lawn and hosed him down with a garden hose for almost five minutes." Chad is starting to learn that I am aggressive, but maybe not as far gone as he thought a thirty-year medic would be. It is simply a matter of time and experience. Having been in the same situation a dozen times, I automatically know what to do and when to do it. I am helping Chad learn, and he is helping me relearn.

Chad and I had some tough calls together, one of which came in as chest pain. When we arrived at the patient's house and brought all of the gear into the patient's bedroom, he was sitting up on his bed with his back against the headboard. His automatic defibrillator was shocking him every minute and he was going in and out of consciousness, so we put him on our EKG monitor. We saw that he was going in and out of ventricular fibrillation. We attempted to defibrillate with our machine, thinking a higher setting would convert him, but we could not time it correctly. The patient went into a bradycardic rhythm, so we switched over to our external pacing which sustained him for about a minute before he stopped breathing and lost pulses. We placed the patient on the floor and the fire department started CPR, Chad intubated the patient while I set him up an IV bag of Normal Saline. After Chad initiated the IV and taped it in place, I handed him a prefilled syringe of Epinephrine 1mg and 1mg of Atropine. The patient remained in a slow pulseless heart rhythm and as we looked at it closer, it was a paced rhythm. Apparently the implanted defibrillator had an intrinsic pacemaker that was not working, and we initially overrode it with or external pace-making attempt. We continued our efforts with no avail until our arrival at the ER, where another ten minutes of resuscitation was of ill effect, the code blue was stopped on the physician's orders.

The next week, we got a difficulty-breathing call that was serious. When we got on-scene, the patient was a 78-year-old male in extreme distress. He was skinny with a barrel chest and the smell of cigarette smoke in the house told us he had emphysema. His lung sounds we decreased bilaterally with mild expiratory wheezes; he was not moving enough air. We started off with an Albuterol nebulizer treatment while getting vital signs and placing the patient on the monitor. The patients pulse oximetry was registering at 79 percent, and as we loaded him into the ambulance, he started getting worse. I set Chad up a bag of Saline and spiked it with fifteen cc IV tubing, while Chad put a tourniquet on the patient's arm to prepare for an IV attempt. I grabbed an Ambu bag and laid it on the bench seat before jumping up front for a code 3 run to the ER. Chad had his hands full with the patient, so I called in a brief radio report to the hospital. I asked how it's going back there and Chad said the patient was crashing, but still too conscious to intubate as he had tried once. I told him we were almost there, and upon arrival I would jump in the back and give him a hand. When we pulled into the ambulance bay, I jumped out and opened the rear doors and saw Chad attempting to assist respirations with an inline nebulizer treatment connected to the Ambu bag. Chad set up for another intubation attempt, but the patient was still too conscious. When Chad was ready with the laryngoscope and ET tube, I laid the patient flat. As Chad was starting to introduce the laryngoscope blade, the charge nurse came out into the ambulance bay yelling at me to get the patient inside. I was sweating like crazy and struggling to help Chad, so I yelled back at her. Chad, knowing the repercussions, stopped and said, "Let's take him in." We wheeled the patient into the ER where they had a room and a doctor waiting, and Chad gave his report. The doctor initiated RSI and successfully gained control of the patient's airway. Back outside we were preparing the gurney and cleaning the back of the unit before restock. Chad told me the charge nurse was livid and was going to write me up. I told Chad that it won't be the first time. Chad, being the good friend and honorable person that he is, told me he was going to go in speak with the charge nurse. I was still steaming, but managed to get myself in check. Knowing that the ER staff was ready and waiting, I was definitely in the wrong, and I put my partner into a bad situation due to my bad judgment. After walking into the room where Chad was explaining to the RN and physician it was his patient and his responsibility, I made apologies and took credit for my poor decision and all was forgiven and forgot.

Chad had just married and, on the next shift bid, moved to day shifts, so he could be home at night with his new bride. Luckily enough, he drew Turp as a partner. They were good friends and there was no EMT I would rather see by Chad's side. This would be a perfect match since Matt was now enrolled in paramedic school.

I still had first choice on shift bids and I prefer nights so I picked my usual 206 unit on the first half of the week, which is 6 p.m. to 6 a.m. I drew Michael Conover for my partner and, while we had never worked together before, we had the same close friends working the streets.

Conover and I started off our first shift by grabbing some dinner at my favorite taco truck Elvia's, on East Avenue. The guys that own and work the truck know me because I always thank them and praise them followed by tip. They like to compensate me with larger portions and extra jalapenos. These are hardworking guys who can make a taco or burrito with just the right amount of grease and salsa to make your mouth water in anticipation. I managed to get Mike to eat at the taco truck every night for three months straight, even though I was almost getting tired of it; I wanted to see how much he could take before saying something.

Finally, after three months, when I asked Mike if he was ready for dinner he caved in and said, "Yeah, anything but taco truck." I laughed and told him I wondered when he would have had enough.

Michael and I loved our jobs so much that we showed up early to wash and stock our unit. Ok we enjoyed our job as medics and working on the street, that we made it the most fun and least stressful as possible. Our Employer only gave negative feedback so Conover and I decided to be all we could be, so instead of feeling negative towards our employer, we decided to do what needed to be done for own integrity, at least for the most part. The company had recently mixed the Turlock units with the Modesto units, so where we used to always stay in town, we were now running back and forth. It was a bitter pill to swallow, as we had different unions and a different contract agreement. The Modesto crews had a higher pay grade and were allowed two 30-minute lunch breaks to our one. They also had VST's (vehicle service technicians) to wash and stock their units, which we did ourselves. The worst part for most, if not all of us, was after logging into the system and going available. We would be posted to whatever area was uncovered. That would usually mean driving into Modesto while two or three Modesto units were covering our area in Turlock. We never had a problem with a slightly lesser wage, stocking, and washing our own units because Turlock was our home and we were familiar with it. Now we were driving around like yo-yos, up and down Hwy 99, shifting posts every time a call came in or a unit wanted a lunch break. All in all, my worst habit was when I was in Turlock and I had a patient who did not warrant transportation and wanted to be transported an extra twenty minutes into a Modesto hospital. I would simply do my best at convincing them that Emanuel Hospital in Turlock is just five minutes away and that is where they should go. Likewise, when in Modesto and a drunk or homeless person would dial 911, knowing that the patient did not need an ambulance or a hospital, I would talk them into the great service they would receive at Emanuel. Being in Turlock for most of thirty years, I found comfort in knowing where we were going when responding to a call, as well as often knowing the patient and their history. We also knew what to expect from the fire department and the police department, as well as the local ER staff. While I had my little tricks to stay in Turlock as much as possible, others had theirs, from taking a lunch break into a slower area, or stacking two lunch breaks together and running them into fuel time.

Conover and I showed up for work early as usual one day and after stocking and cleaning our unit, we logged on and immediately received a code 3 call at Fulkerth and Countryside roads, across the street from Wal-Mart, for a vehicle vs. a four year old pedestrian. We went en-route with dispatch and hauled ass over there, faster than normal, as no medic wants harm to come to a child. When we pulled up alongside the fire truck blocking the East bound three lanes, we saw the firemen c-collaring a young female adult to a long back board. We both get out and asked at the same time, "Where is the 4 year-old?" The firemen answered that this was the only patient. She was twenty-four years old, per their dispatch. I walked over and bent down, checking the patient's wrist for a radial pulse only to find that was present and strong. I asked the firemen if the patient was speaking and they said she was not. I gave her a strong sternal rub, which she did not respond to. The firemen advise me that the driver of the car is o.k., and that she said the patient was struck at about thirty miles an hour and flew ten feet, striking her head.

I asked the fire department to cut her clothes off and continue with the spinal immobilization as Conover to my side with the trauma bag. I asked him to pull out the airway kit and an Ambu bag while I advise the fire department that I am going to intubate the patient, and I will need one fireman to assist respirations. With laryngoscope and an 8.0 ET tube in hand, I was able to quickly insert the tube past the patient's vocal cords. I asked Mike to secure the tube as I confirmed placement by auscultation. With one fireman now assisting ventilations, I asked Conover to have the fire department load the patient into the ambulance when they are done. "I want you, Mike, to set me up two lines of Saline in the back of the unit and tear me some tape. I am going to do a trauma alert on the med-net to Doctor's Hospital and we are going to rock and roll." I called Doctor's Medical Center in Modesto and when they answered I told them, "We are currently on-scene with a 24 year old female, auto vs. pedestrian, who appears to have an isolated open-skull fracture to the left parietal skull. The patient is intubated and almost fully immobilized. We should see you in less than twenty minutes." The hospital replied, "We copy, I think you have to go through Stanislaus Control for a destination."

I replied, "Negative. This is code 3 and you are the closest receiving trauma facility. I will update you en-route." We had been on-scene about eight minutes and as I walked to the back of the ambulance, the fire department was starting to load the patient. I jumped in the back and Mike asked what I needed. I answered, "I've got it. Haul ass to Doctor's ER." I had one fireman assisting ventilations while I got a blood pressure of 134/88 and a pulse rate of 84. I hooked the patient up to the EKG monitor which showed a sinus rhythm corresponding with pulses at 84 bpm. Next, I attached the capnography to the ET tube and saw a nice wave pattern confirming proper tube placement. As we rolled onto Hwy 99, I slid in my first IV, quickly followed by a second in the opposite arm. Both IVs were TKO as I reexamined the patient's pupils, which were midpoint and sluggish. The only trauma I could see was the apparent open-skull fracture. The fact that it was open and not closed was probably why the patient was still alive. Most often with a closed head injury, the cerebral pressure increases, causing coma and then death. I called on the med-net radio to update the hospital with a current ETA. Everything was under control with the patient so having another few minutes; I spiked a third bag of Norma Saline and started an extra third IV with a 16ga angio catheter for good measure. We arrived at Doctor's Medical Center and prepared to unload the patient where a trauma team was awaiting us. While we don't always have a chance to follow up with patients, we did check back the next day to find out that the young woman had expired that morning.

I had been involved in some court litigation where the company had pulled me off the ambulance during my shift. I'd had a cervical fusion in 2006 and, after a six-month recovery, had returned back to work. I had been back at work for 14 months without incident when the workers compensation carrier challenged the QME (qualified medical expert) and he, in turn, placed a prophylactic lifting restriction of 100 pounds on my revised report. I was on-duty and had no idea about this new restriction. I was in the ambulance posting in Turlock when I received a phone call from the acting Human Resource Director. I was told to take myself out of service and contact my attorney. While we were having the conversation, I asked what I need to do to come to work tomorrow. The reply was, have your doctor give you a no lift restriction. Our unit was dispatched to a code

3 call while on the phone, I asked if I should take the call or go out of service? I was told to run the call and then take myself out of service. It was about 4 p.m., so I called my doctor's office while we were rolling code 3. Luckily, they all know me on a first name basis, and I requested an emergency visit. Of course, the call was a serious respiratory distress and a code 3 in transport. In the end, I was able to take care of the patient and make it to the doctor's office just before closing. I was evaluated and asked if my neurosurgeon had released me to work. I said yes and that I had been back for 14 months without a problem. Returning to work the next day with my release in hand and not knowing at this time any restriction had ever been placed, I was told that the QME had to give me the release. I was off work for about 5 months, fighting to get my job back. I had to endure several FCE's (functional capacity exams) before being allowed to return. Meanwhile, I was in my second year of owning and running Mr. Slice Pizza, a business I bought as an exit strategy. I was finally just breaking even and moving ahead when I lost my paramedic income, which helped me support my restaurant. I lost the business, filed suit against my employer, and won the case in a three-week courtroom battle. AMR had considered me disabled and had not attempted to engage in a verbal reconciliation or any attempt to accommodate me, if in fact I needed it, which I did not. This was a violation of Fair Employment Act.

Returning to work on the 206 unit, Michael and I were back on the street. We ate dinner at the taco truck and had run a few of the usual calls when we got dispatched to 55 year-old male with CPR in progress. When we rolled our gurney and equipment into the house, we found the fire department having just got there a minute ahead of us, performing CPR. The local EMS agency had recently changed our protocols and preferred we start an IV first if the patient was not in ventricular fibrillation. In fact, the new guidelines wanted us to consider intubation en-route to the hospital. I could understand the rationale for this under controlled settings as in the hospital, but not in the field. I don't believe you can have a secure airway doing CPR from the patient's bedroom and out into the hallway and then onto the gurney, followed by walking out to the ambulance. The time it takes to start an IV, especially if you miss the first shot is much greater than dropping an ET tube. I also felt that in order to properly ventilate the patient, it takes two people: one to hold a seal on the mask and another to ventilate with an Ambu bag. By the time my partner places the patient on the EKG monitor and has a line spiked for an IV, I will have the airway done and be waiting to start the IV.

I had Conover place the defibrillation pads (which also act as EKG pads) to show me the rhythm, followed by spiking a line of Normal Saline solution. I grabbed the laryngoscope with a Macintosh number 4 blade, an 8.0 ET tube, a ten cc syringe, and cloth tape before getting myself into position. Conover had the patient attached to the pads, so I asked to hold CPR and checked the rhythm. It was a sinus rhythm at 82 bpm, I checked for a carotid pulse that was not there, meaning the patient was in PEA (pulseless electrical activity). Having the firemen continue CPR, I intubated the patient and confirmed placement, followed by filling the pilot balloon with 10 cc's of air and then securing the tube aggressively with tape. I dropped 2mg. of Epinephrine down the tube while Mike hooked the capnography up to the ET tube and we were looking good.

Mike had the IV ready to go so I grabbed a 14ga catheter and slide it into the patient's left external jugular vein. Mike handed me a preload of Epinephrine and I administered another milligram through the IV. I had the IV running wide open since the patient did not appear to have any CHF (congestive heart failure) components. We were not getting any kind of medical history on the patient because he was on the phone with his daughter when he went down and she called 911. I drew up 10 mg of Epinephrine 1:10,000 into the 10cc syringe I kept from inflating the ET tube, and I now had a convenient way to administer the medication in 1mg increments with the IV running wide open. The patient remained in PEA with CPR being continued as I administered another mg of epinephrine. We were getting ready to load the patient when I noticed some type of J-peg in the patient's abdomen. These can sometimes be used for retroperitoneal dialysis in patients who aren't bad enough to need standard dialysis. They simply pump Normal Saline in and out of their gut daily to decreases the potassium content. With this in mind, I asked Mike to hand me a box of Calcium Chloride and I administered 1000 mgs IV. After loading the patient into the ambulance and twenty-minutes of CPR, we noticed the patient was trying to breathe on his own. Stopping CPR, we found a nice strong radial pulse and got a blood pressure of 140/82. When we arrived at Emanuel ER, the patient had is eyes open and would squeeze my hands upon request. We transported patient care over to Emanuel ER and started about the business of putting our car back together. When we were done, I asked Mike if he was ready. He asked, "Ready for what?" "To go home", I said, "I think this is about as good as it gets; let's go have some Crown at my house." He replied, "Let's do it." I called the supervisor, who was Holly that evening, and told her we were going home. She asked, "Are you guys too stressed out to finish your shift?" I replied, "No, we just saved a patient and want to go home on a good note for a change to celebrate." Holly laughed and said she would meet us at the station. Off to the liquor store, then my house. It was time for Crown Royale and tall tales.

Back on shift and working the night, we found ourselves in a crappy part of Modesto. We had already found every good taco truck in the county. The ones in Crows Landing were often open until 2 a.m. and one of them used barbequed tri-tip. Eating at the taco truck helped to lessen the pain of working in Modesto. After trying out our new found cuisine and running a few calls, we realized that some of the nursing staff at the Modesto hospitals were starting to trust our judgment, and not only that, but a lot of them were easy on the eyes.

Mike and I were responded to a supposed respiratory distress call in the unincorporated, and generally more dangerous, part of Modesto. When we arrived, we saw several Modesto firemen and family members crowded around a figure lying out on the front lawn. Mike and I shook our heads, assuming this to be another alcohol or drug-related problem, but we were wrong. As I got out of the ambulance with my stethoscope around my neck, Mikes grabbed the medical bag off the gurney and we walked together to see what was going on. The patient was 30 years-old with a history of asthma. She started having trouble breathing and her MDI (metered dose inhaler) ran out. It was dark outside, and I could barely see well enough to realize this was the real deal; the patient appeared to be moving very little air. I listened for lung sounds and could only hear a slight, expiratory wheeze. I asked Mike for an Ambu bag and hooked it up to the firemen's oxygen.

They call asthma the silent killer because it can come on quickly and sometimes can't be reversed in time. Our patient was unconscious and not responsive to verbal or painful stimuli. I had Michael draw me up .3 mg of Epinephrine as I directed the firemen to assist ventilations. As Conover handed me the medication, I asked him to set me up for an intubation. I injected the Epinephrine subcutaneously into the female's left shoulder. I grabbed the laryngoscope, a 7.0 ET tube, a 10cc syringe to fill the pilot balloon, and some tape. As I attempted to insert the blade into the patient's mouth, I realized her jaw was clamped shut. I should have checked that first. I asked Conover to go to the unit and set up an inline albuterol treatment; I told him I would be right there with the patient. The fire department guys helped me load the patient onto the gurney and into the ambulance where Michael was waiting. I asked for one fireman to ride along and assist with ventilations, and I asked Michael for lights and sirens to Memorial Medical Center. I shouted up front to Conover "I love you man," Just to break the stress a little. Conover replied back, "I love you too, wimp." I connected the inline nebulizer filled with Albuterol and hooked it into a separate oxygen source then attached it to the bag valve mask that the fireman was using to ventilate. At times like these, I have to sometimes leave the protocols behind and do what I feel is right and what I have experienced to be in the patient's best interest (in this case it was holding off on the pulse oximetry and vitals and starting treatment first). Attaching the pulse oximetry now, and getting a reading of 84% saturation, I was not surprised. A blood pressure gave me 158/84 and the monitor was, of course, sinus tachycardia at 140 bpm. That was also not a surprise, considering all of the Epinephrine and continuous Albuterol treatments. Ordinarily I would attempt a nasal intubation, but the county EMS agency (in its great wisdom, or lack of in this case) removed it from our scope of practice after introducing CPAP. Using CPAP is contraindicated for patients who are unconscious, so the patient needed to have a RSI (rapid sequence intubation). In the old days, aggressive paramedics would snow the patient with a rapid IV push of Valium, but they got wise to our tricks and started pulling paramedic patches. Now I have to be a little more creative if my patients are going to live.

I called Memorial Medical Center on the med-net radio and gave give them a heads-up code 3 report, while spiking a line of Normal Saline. Asthma patients need lots of fluid to help break up mucus that is accumulating in their air sacks from the release of histamine receptors. I actually had just enough time to slip in two 18 ga angio catheters and TKO (to keep open) the second IV line, while I let the first one dump 500 cc's of fluid before reassessing my patient's condition. The patient was still unconscious and unresponsive and her pupils were midpoint and reactive--which was good. The pulse oximetry had barely moved up two points at 86% saturation. I thought to myself, *if I was up in Arnold I would have to administer whatever amount Valium or Versed necessary to this patient to take over their airway, or I would be doing CPR thirty minutes before arriving at an emergency room.* Of course, I might have to give up my career, but that's just how it is; you have to treat every patient like family. When we arrived at Memorial Medical Center in Modesto, we were immediately ushered by security into a high-priority room. I gave my full report to the physician and apologized for the patient not being intubated because we did not have RSI guidelines and the local EMS authority recently took away nasal intubation. The physician and nurses worked fast to RSI the patient and continue ventilations with an inline albuterol treatment. The patient's blood gasses were horrendous, but in the end she managed to pull through after spending several days in the ICU.

Mike and I cleaned and restocked the ambulance to ready ourselves for the next medical aid. I was a little frustrated that we could not do more, and felt that when a new tool such as CPAP is introduced, the old tools should not be taken away because you never know when a need may arise. It was going on 5 a.m. when we got cleared back to Turlock for fuel and then we cleared off-duty. It was Wednesday night of our long week, so we would partake in our normal, twice-a-month ritual. We cleared with dispatch and clocked out. We went to the liquor store that opens right at 6 a.m., which was pretty convenient, despite the fact that the personnel working there always asked if we are on are way into work. Of course, Conover replied, "We don't start until 7 a.m.; don't forget to buckle up now." Michael and I rolled over to my residence for Crown Royale on ice, and another rare victory dance.

On Saturday afternoon, Mike was having his son's third birthday party and a barbeque. His fiancée, Haley, who was in nursing school, had bought Crown and Michael told me that it is for me. He had cooked up five gallons of a family recipe of chili and beans that were awesome, and we followed the afternoon into dusk with a bon-fire and laughter.

Back on duty Sunday night at 6 p.m., and we took a change from taco truck, and we grabbed sandwiches at Subway. We ran a couple of routine calls in Turlock before getting sent to Modesto for coverage. We were kind of hoping for a quit shift because we were a little hung over from Saturday night's birthday party. As luck would have it, we got called for a two-victim shooting. When we arrived, there was another ambulance already on-scene, and it was reported that there was one gunshot victim in each of the two houses which sat next door to each other. We took the house closest to our unit, pulled out our gurney with the med bag on it and headed in. A sheriff's officer was waving us forward telling us that there was one patient inside and that the area was secure. We found a 22 year-old Hispanic male with two gunshot wounds to his chest. I reached down for a radial pulse and asked the victim how many times he had been shot. His radial pulse was faint, thready, and rapid--not good. Conover cut his shirt and we found two entrance wounds in his right upper chest. Rolling him over, we saw that there were no exit wounds. The patient's lung sounds were clear and equal, which was a relief, however the patient had lost his bowels, and that did not smell very good. Every medic has their weakness and mine is olfactory. We striped his pants and underwear off to help as much as possible with the stench, and we loaded him onto the gurney with a non-rebreather mask at high flow. I sent Mike out to spike me two lines of Saline while I negotiated getting the patient on the gurney and out to the unit. The fire department had taken a blood pressure that was 84/60 and a heart rate of 140 bpm, there was no external uncontrolled bleeding. We had been on-scene less than five minutes when Mike started us for Memorial Medical Center, code 3. Conover had my two bags of Saline ready to go, and I brought one fireman along for good measure. I put him to work placing the EKG monitor on the patient and I prepared to start my first IV. Mike told me we were ten minutes out, so I asked him to notify the ER of our ETA on the med-net. I shouted the patient's vitals and condition to him up in the front of the cab. As luck would have It, I dropped my second 14ga in the patient's left ac and put it at TKO since I had the first one running wide open. We still had five minutes to our arrival so I decided to set myself up a third line of Saline and sank a 16ga angio-catheter in the patient's left wrist. The first IV bag of solution was almost gone, so I changed it out for a fresh one and made a mental note to pass that on to the ER staff. We pulled into the hospital and security was waiting for us, directing us into the main trauma room. As we transferred the patient over to their bed from our gurney, I ascertained which doctor was in charge as there were three physicians, as well as three nurses, awaiting us. I only wanted to have to give my report once, so I gave my report to the head trauma physician. I heard one of the doctors ask a nurse to start another IV line and she quickly replied, "The paramedics have already got three large bore IVs in place." Before Mike and I could get out of the ER, the trauma team had already started transfusing blood through a pump. The doctors had ultrasound equipment out and an x-ray machine rolling in. I walked over to a fourth nurse who was sitting down, charting, and told her, "You folks are flat-out fantastic; thanks for being ready for us." Conover and I walked back out to the unit and started in on the cleanup. There was no need for restock because Mike and I were always stocked up to the breach, just in case of calls like this.

On our next tour, the night shift went slowly as we worked our way up and down Hwy 99 between twenty-two miles of posts from Turlock to Salida. Stopping for post assignments and felling like a ping pong ball, we finally settled into Hatch and Herndon in Ceres for about an hour.

As the hour wound down, we were responded code 3 to a man down in the McDonalds parking lot. When we rolled up, it was 3:30 in the morning when Mike pulled to a stop. I saw a transient lying in the shrubbery waving and yelling.
I rolled my window down and heard him yelling, "I'm over here, man."
"Ok, I see you, shut up." I told Mike to stay put as I jumped out to see what was causing all the commotion. "It's my ankle man,

it's my ankle."

"What happened," I asked.

"I twisted it three months ago and it hurts; I need to go to the hospital."

I replied "Can you stand up and walk?"

"Oh yea, man, I can walk. They call me Mad Dog."

"All right, mad man, I mean, Mad Dog, here's the deal. My partner and I are on our way back to Turlock, so if it's o.k., we will give you a ride there."

Mad Dog replied, "Oh hell yes, man. Cool." I waved for Michael to get out and he walked over to me, as I explained that we were going to help Mad Dog out by taking him to the hospital in Turlock. Conover took him to the ambulance and had him climb into the back. Meanwhile, I had noticed that there were no cars in the Macdonald's drive-thru and the drive through window was open with the employee hanging out it, watching the action and shaking his head. I walked over, ordered 3 cheese burgers, and carried them back to the unit. I threw one to Mad Dog and one to Mike as I headed to the driver's door of the ambulance, jumping in with my own burger in tow. The patient was yelling, "You guys are the greatest crew I have ever called. Can you turn on the sirens?" I said, "No problem, yelp, yelp." We dropped Mad Dog off in the triage area of the hospital where the entire room was packed with walk-in patients. We gave report to the nurse, who then started laughing like crazy. Conover and I went back in service and caught a Turlock post. We drove over to the Chevron on Geer and Regis, jumped out of the unit, and grabbed a complimentary soda as we both laughed about Mad Dog. An hour went by before we were toned out for a man with ankle pain across the street at the Raley's phone booth. We pulled in and the Mad Dog was waving like crazy again. When he saw that it was us, he started laughing and laughing.

Conover asked, "What's up, Dog? You are supposed to be at the hospital."

"Yea man, the wait was too long. Can you take me back?"

"No problem." I said as I jumped out and piled into the back of the ambulance with him drove back to the hospital triage waiting area. Michael and I had about twenty minutes each of reports to write on Mad Dog, but it was worth it because he was so funny and he was actually very appreciative.

We got cleared for fuel and were heading for the station a couple of hours later when we spotted a man on the side of the road waving us over. Yep, it was the Mad Dog. I rolled down the window and he was grinning ear to ear. He told us to take him to the bus station. Mad Dog jumped into the back of the unit before we could say a word, and Mike and I laughed as we hit the siren a couple times on our way to the bus station. Mad Dog jumped out of the unit at the bus depot and thanked us. We each handed him a fiver and told him we would see him next shift.

NOTE:

To all the new medical personnel starting your new professions, please remember that while the calls and patient treatment in this book are true, I would not recommend you to ever deviate from your established guidelines. With time you will figure out your own recipe for success.

About the Author

After spending 30 years on the streets of the Central Valley and Mountains of California, Paramedic William Coakley wrote his first book, *Still of Darkness*.

Bill worked as a law enforcement officer in Tuolumne and Calaveras counties for 6 years in boat patrol services before deciding to become a paramedic. He has owned several businesses including Valley Springs Ambulance with his partners Bill Macfall and Robert Easter as well as owning and operating, Mr.Slice Pizza in Turlock.

Bill has also received several patents pending and 1 patent in 1995.

Find out more about Bill @ billcoakley.com

Like Bill'sFacebookpage:

https://www.facebook.com/pages/ Bill-Coakley Authors page/680077895349124

Bill would love to hear from you, leave feedback and a review on the book at Amazon.com

www.ingramcontent.com/pod-product-compliance
Lightning Source LLC
Chambersburg PA
CBHW061729020426
42331CB00006B/1155